# Conditioning for Soccer

## Joseph A. Luxbacher

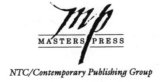

MASTERS PRESS

NTC/Contemporary Publishing Group

**Library of Congress Cataloging-in-Publication Data**

Luxbacher, Joe.
    Conditioning for soccer / Joseph A. Luxbacher.
        p.    cm.
    Includes bibliographical references (p.).
    ISBN 1-57028-146-7
    1. Soccer—Training.   2. Soccer—Physiological aspects.   I. Title.
GV943.9.T7L886    1997
796.334—dc21                                97-30050
                                                        CIP

Cover design by Christy Pierce
Cover photographs by Steve Parker
Diagrams by Suzanne Lincoln
Editorial Assistants: Pat Brady and Matt Witten

Published by Masters Press
A division of NTC/Contemporary Publishing Group, Inc.
4255 West Touhy Avenue, Lincolnwood (Chicago), Illinois 60712-1975 U.S.A.
Copyright © 1997 by Joseph A. Luxbacher
Printed in the United States of America
International Standard Book Number: 1-57028-146-7
    01  02  03  04  05  BG  21  20  19  18  17  16  15  14  13  12  11  10  9  8  7  6  5

# Table of Contents

# Acknowledgments

The writing and publishing of a book takes a team effort. I am greatly indebted to a number of individuals for their help and cooperation in bringing this project to fruition. Although it is not possible to mention everyone by name, I would like to express my deepest appreciation to the following individuals.

√   The outstanding staff at Masters Press, particularly Tom Bast and Holly Kondras, for their confidence in this project.

√   Leslie Bonci, Food and Nutrition expert, for her willingness to share information concerning eating for peak performance. Leslie is a media spokesperson for the American Dietetic Association. Her clients include the University of Pittsburgh Athletic Department, the Pittsburgh Ballet Theater, and the Pittsburgh Steelers Football Team.

√   Gary Wateska, Strength and Conditioning Coach at the University of Pittsburgh, for development of the strength and conditioning programs listed in Chapters 5 and 12. Gary has formerly worked with the Pittsburgh Steelers (NFL) and Pittsburgh

Penguins (NHL).

√   Chris Karwoski, assistant men's soccer coach at the University of Pittsburgh, for his assistance in organizing many of the drills and exercises.

√   Jason Anstead, Phil Matilla, and Scott Pine, for their help with the demonstration of the strength training and flexibility exercises.

√   Photographer Les Banos for taking the photos used in Chapters 6 and 8.

Special thanks goes to my mother, Mary Ann Luxbacher, for her love and support of everything that I do. Most importantly, I would like to thank my beautiful wife Gail for her constant love, support and patience, particularly when the writing deadlines drew near. She, along with our daughter Eliza Gail, are a constant source of inspiration.

# Preface

*"Fitness can neither be bought nor bestowed. Like honor, it must be earned."*

Soccer may be the most demanding of all team sports. The game is played on the largest field area of any sport except polo (where horses do most of the work!), for the longest sustained time with the least breaks in play. A typical game consists of ninety minutes of virtually nonstop action, because substitutions are limited and there are no official time outs. Field players may run more than six miles during the course of a match, often at sprint intensity. A player's level of fitness is a critical factor affecting his or her ability to successfully cope with the physical demands of the match.

There is an old coaching adage that states " fitness is not everything, but without fitness you have nothing". This statement rings particularly true for the game of soccer where a number of variables interact to determine a player's level of performance. A high level of fitness , although important, in and of itself will not guarantee superior performance on the soccer field. The ability to execute skills and make split-second decisions under the pressures of game competition, coupled with a thorough knowledge of individual, group and team tactics, is equally important. All other things being equal, however, the player who is more physically fit can potentially achieve higher levels of performance and sustain that performance for longer periods of time. So, while it may be true that fitness is not everything, it is also true that a player's level of physical conditioning provides the foundation upon which other elements of performance are based. That being the case, we can guarantee with utmost certainty that a player's potential for elite soccer performance can be dramatically improved through comprehensive fitness training.

To achieve a high level of soccer-specific fitness, players must have knowledge of the physical demands imposed upon them. They must identify important fitness goals and then devise a step-by-step plan to achieve those goals. In other words, players must know "what to do and how to do it." *Conditioning For Soccer is* written with that theme in mind. The following pages provide players and coaches with a practical step-by-step guide for achieving total soccer fitness. Proven training methods used to develop aerobic and anaerobic endurance, muscular strength and power, flexibility and agility are examined in detail. Guidelines for optimal nutrition and fluid replacement are also provided. Each of these fitness components impact overall performance to varying degrees.

The ultimate goal of this book is to prepare soccer players to more successfully cope with the physical challenges they will encounter during match play, and to ensure that their technical and tactical abilities are utilized to the fullest extent for the entire 90 minutes of each game. Keep in mind, however, that no one is born with a high level of fitness. It must be earned through diligent effort and hard work. So, while this book provides a blueprint for achieving total soccer fitness, the individual player must provide the determination and persistence required to make any good plan work. There are no shortcuts to success.

*Joseph A. Luxbacher*
*Pittsburgh, Pennsylvania*
*June 30, 1997*

# Conditioning
# for Soccer

# 1 Physiological Demands

A soccer match is characterized by continuous, sub-maximal effort interspersed with periods of shorter-term, high intensity activity. Players are in constant motion as they contest for loose balls, move to support teammates, interchange positions, and run to create space or track opponents. Running, jumping, and sprinting movements in tandem with sudden changes of speed and direction dominate the play.

The intensity of exercise ranges between low level activities like walking, jogging and cruising and those of higher intensity, like maximal effort sprint running. The rhythm of play is constantly changing, a characteristic that separates soccer from other types of endurance sports where the intensity of activity remains relatively stable throughout the competition. The physiological demands imposed upon players are great and vary with respect to the level of competition, playing style, positional roles and responsibilities, and environmental factors.

One method of estimating work load is to determine how far a player runs during a game. The total distance covered provides an approximate representation of energy expenditure as well as the overall severity of the exercise. Numerous studies have used motion analysis methods in an effort to quantify player movements during a game. Activity is generally categorized according to type, intensity, duration, and frequency. There has been considerable variance in the results of these studies, although many of the inconsistencies are due in part to the differing styles of play and levels of competition of the teams in question. Most studies indicate that field players average between 9 and 12 km (5.6 to 7.5 miles) during a typical 90-minute game. The total distance covered can be subdivided into walking, jogging, cruising, sprinting, backward and sideward movement. Combining results from independent studies (Table 1.1 Nike Research Review) provides a more complete picture of player movement patterns. These findings lead to the conclusion that field players should develop a sufficient level of aerobic fitness to enable them to run 6 or more miles in relatively continuous fashion. Of particular interest is the revelation that less than 2% of the distance covered by a field player during a game is "with the ball". The vast majority of physical effort is actually performed "off (without) the ball" as players run in support of teammates, to create space, or to track opponents.

The total distance covered during a game actually underestimates energy expenditure because it fails to account for the extra efforts needed to perform skills. Not only must players run several miles, but they do so while executing tackles, headers, shots at goal, and dribbling maneuvers. Added to these movements are

## Table 1.1 Player Movement Patterns

|  | Total | Standing | Walking | Jogging | Cruising | Sprinting | W/ Ball |
|---|---|---|---|---|---|---|---|
| Distance (meters) | 10,000 | NA | 2600 | 4900 | 1700 | 800 | 180 |
| Distance (% of total) | 100 | NA | 26 | 49 | 17 | 8 | <2 |

* Taken from Nike Sport Research Review, Volume No.5, 1997

numerous other actions such as turns, jumps, accelerations and decelerations. Although the energy cost and effort of isolated actions is relatively small, the total aggregate of such actions requires substantial effort above and beyond the total distance covered. In short, the more active a player is the more energy he or she will expend. Or, from a different point of view, a more physically fit player is likely to be more active than a less fit player over the course of a 90-minute match.

## Factors Affecting a Player's Work load

A number of aspects can influence the physiological demands required of a player during a game. The following discussion examines a few of these factors.

### POSITIONAL ROLE WITHIN THE TEAM

Studies comparing activity levels by position have revealed what most coaches and players would probably expect. Midfielders generally cover the greatest distances, central defenders the least, with strikers and flank defenders falling somewhere in-between. Results of independent studies are summarized in Table 1.2. Goalkeepers are excluded in this analysis.

The type and intensity of running also varies from one position to another. The greater overall distance covered by midfielders was generally due to more running at low intensities, a pace sometimes referred to as cruising. Central defenders devote a higher percentage of their movement going backward and sideways than do strikers and flank defenders. Studies of English League players have revealed that the overall

| Table 1.2 Distance (meters) Covered During a Soccer Game Broken Down by Position | | | | | |
|---|---|---|---|---|---|
| | Total | Walk | Jog | Cruise | Sprint | W/ Ball |
| Midfield | 11040 | 2340 | 5760 | 2040 | 900 | 230 |
| Fullback | 10000 | 2550 | 4930 | 1660 | 860 | 190 |
| Striker | 10000 | 2850 | 4730 | 1520 | 900 | 160 |
| Centerback | 8960 | 2360 | 4480 | 1470 | 650 | 160 |

\* Distances were based on an average of 10 km games for fullbacks and strikers
\*\* Taken from Nike Sport Research Review, Volume No.5, 1997

distance covered sprinting was significantly less for both fullbacks and central defenders than for strikers and midfielders. Sprinting runs by the strikers included decoy or "dummy" runs designed to draw opponents into poor defensive positions, as well as inadvertent offside runs that were not followed by a defender.

For those who believe that the goalkeeper need not be concerned with developing aerobic fitness, they may be surprised to learn that keepers may cover as much as 4 km (2.4 miles) during the course of a game. Much of this movement is in the form of walking, jogging, and moving backward.

## AEROBIC FITNESS LEVEL

An individual's activity profile, or how active he or she is over the course of a match, is determined in part by his or her level of aerobic fitness. Aerobic fitness is usually measured in terms of oxygen uptake ability, referred to as VO2 max. Oxygen uptake can be measured quite easily in the laboratory setting. It is difficult, however, if not impossible, to get a realistic value for VO2 max during a game because it would interfere with normal play. Fortunately a reliable estimate of VO2 max can be obtained by measuring a player's heart rate (HR) during exercise. Heart rate can be monitored with little restriction on the player, so it represents a more reliable estimate of the aerobic demands incurred during actual competition. Based upon numerous studies, it is estimated that competitive match play requires an average oxygen uptake of 75% of VO2 max. This value reflects an effort level comparable with that experienced in marathon running. Studies of higher level performers also demonstrate that midfield players, who generally shoulder the heaviest work load during the match, possess the highest values for aerobic capacity. Flank defenders and strikers demonstrate intermediate values while central defenders tend to have the lowest. These findings are consistent with what one would expect based on positional roles and responsibilities.

## FATIGUE

Work rate is also affected by a player's level of fatigue, which in turn can be linked to the individual's level of fitness. Obviously, a more fit player can sustain higher intensity activity for a longer period of time without a drop-off in performance. This appears to be an increasingly important concern during the latter stages of a game. Motion studies tend to show a general decline in work rate towards the end of a game at all levels of competition. Studies of English League professional games show that in the majority of matches players covered a greater distance during the first half of play as compared to the second half. Similar findings have been reported for Dutch League matches, with a 5% greater distance being covered in the first half. It is also noteworthy to mention that an analysis of goals scored in three divisions of the Scottish League during the 1991-92 season revealed that more goals are scored towards the latter stages of a game than at any other time (See Table 1.3). Obviously this finding cannot be attributed entirely to a decline in work rate, but it does make for interesting discussion.

The onset of physical fatigue may also be linked to a player's nutritional state prior to competition. Muscular glycogen stores available at the beginning of a match seem to influence not only the distance covered during a game but also the type of

## Table 1.3

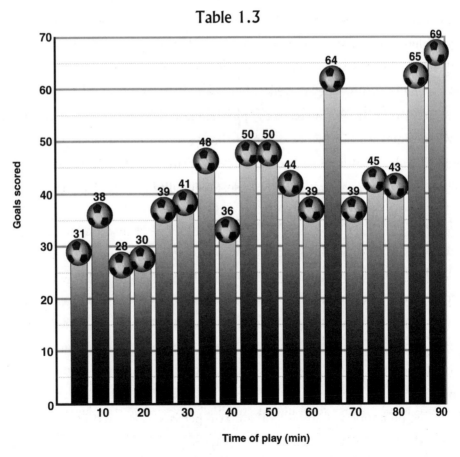

Table 1.3: Goals Scored in Scottish League football during the major part of the 1991-1992 season. * Taken from Handbook of Sport Medicine and Science (Soccer) International Olympic Committee (1994)

running. Several studies have shown that players with low levels of muscle glycogen covered more distance walking and did less sprinting than players with adequate stores of muscle glycogen. Nutritional guidelines for peak soccer performance will be discussed in depth in Chapter 10.

## COMPETITIVE AND ENVIRONMENTAL FACTORS

The level of competition as well as the environmental conditions under which the game is played will also affect the work-rate profiles of players. Aerobic and anaerobic fitness demands tend to increase in concert with the competitive performance level. At the youth (amateur) level, where speed and intensity of play is somewhat less than the professional standard, players may be able to perform adequately with a minimal standard of fitness. As the level of competition improves, however, so must a player's level of fitness. Without the aerobic capacity required to run off-the-ball for extended periods of time, players will be unable to successfully compete at the highest levels where the majority of running (98%) is done without the ball.

Weather conditions will also affect a player's ability to sustain effort over the duration of a match. Games played in hot, humid conditions, such as the matches played in World Cup '94, increase the physiological demands imposed on players. Dehydration and heat exhaustion become potential problems. Likewise, games played at high altitude can also impact performance. Maximum oxygen uptake is impaired which in turn affects a player's ability to sustain quality performance.

## STYLE OF PLAY

A team's style of play will also influence the work rate of its players. Prior to the 1970s, player roles and responsibilities were far more restricted than they are today. Defenders were expected to defend, forwards were expected to score goals, and never the two should meet! All that changed, however, with the onset of "total football." Introduced by the Dutch National Team during their highly successful run during the 1974 World Cup, this highly attractive, attacking style of play placed a premium on player mobility and interchanging of positions. Eleven players attack, eleven defend. The philosophy of "total football" still persists today, and has dramatically increased the fitness requirements of field players.

Cultural factors also influence a team's style of play. The "direct method" of play characteristic of the English League places emphasis on quick movement of the ball from defense to attack through the use of one or two long passes. To the casual observer the game may seem to be played at a frantic pace, and sometimes it is! The direct style of play places extreme demands on aerobic fitness as players are expected to quickly support the ball as it moves from one area of the field to another. At the opposite end of the continuum is the slower paced "South American" style that places greater premium on skill and short interpassing to move the ball forward into goal scoring positions. The so-called European or Continental style combines elements of both the South American and English game. Irrespective of playing style, the most successful teams in major international championships share a common characteristic – the ability of their players to assume a high work load and at the same time maintain a high level of skill throughout the competition. This style of play is best exemplified by the German national teams of the 1980s and 1990s.

## Conclusion

Ideally, players should be able to maintain a consistent level of effort throughout an entire game. For a variety of reasons, fitness being a most critical one, most players find this difficult to do. Physiological demands vary with the level of competition, positional roles and responsibilities, environmental factors, and playing style. Nevertheless, the modern game requires players to develop higher levels of fitness than ever before. They must also demonstrate greater versatility, be able to play more games in a shorter period of time, and be able to play at a higher tempo.

> The modern game requires players to develop higher levels of fitness than ever before.

Soccer players are bigger, faster and, for the most part, better than in the past. The challenge facing coaches and players is to develop an optimal level of fitness without neglecting other aspects of performance. Improvements in fitness must always be accompanied by a corresponding increase in a player's ability to execute skills and make intelligent decisions under the pressures of game competition. In the final analysis it is the movement of the ball, rather than the aggregate distance covered during a game, that distinguishes top level soccer from everything below it. Although players at the highest levels of competition undoubtedly display the highest levels of fitness, they are also the best at making the ball do the work for them. We should never neglect skill for fitness, and the reverse is true as well.

# 2 Training Methods and Myths

The ultimate goals of fitness training are to enable players to successfully cope with the physiological demands of soccer and to ensure that their technical and tactical abilities are used to the fullest extent for the duration of a match. Important components of soccer-related fitness include flexibility and agility, aerobic and anaerobic endurance, muscular strength, muscular endurance, and power. A comprehensive fitness program should address each of these elements.

Include a ball in your fitness workouts whenever possible. Com-

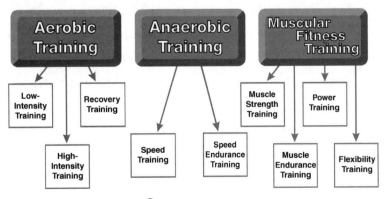

Aerobic Training → Low-Intensity Training, Recovery Training, High-Intensity Training

Anaerobic Training → Speed Training, Speed Endurance Training

Muscular Fitness Training → Muscle Strength Training, Power Training, Muscle Endurance Training, Flexibility Training

bining skill and tactical development with fitness training is the most efficient and effective use of practice time, and it allows players to develop skills and tactics under the physical stressors encountered in a match. The presence of a ball also serves as a motivational factor because, as every soccer player will attest, it is more fun to run after a ball than it is to run laps around the field.

Obviously you won't be able to include a ball in everything that you do. Strength training exercises that utilize free weights and dumbbells, as well as plyometric "jump" training, are cases in point. There are also times when training to improve aerobic and anaerobic capacity, where the emphasis must be solely on fitness, usually because you may not be able to work hard enough when training with a ball to achieve the desired fitness outcomes. In addition, factors not directly related to the activity itself can serve to lower the exercise intensity. For example, the player who is very skillful and clever probably won't have to work as hard to achieve the same results as a less talented individual. To compensate you can increase the physical demands for all players by adding restrictions to the drill. For example, players competing in a 3 versus 3 possession game can be forced to cover more ground by simply increasing the size of the field area. From a fitness standpoint, however, there will be times when it is necessary to train without the ball to maximize the training load.

## Fitness Training for Youth Players

Fitness training is not and should not be a priority with youth players. Rather than spend valuable practice time trying to maximize a 10 year old's level of aerobic endurance, the focus of training should center around skill development. A soccer ball should be included in all drills and game-related exercises. Kids will develop an adequate level of fitness through routine participation in practices and games, and if they aren't superfit, that is okay too. It is much more important for young players to become confident and comfortable with the ball. Besides, preadolescent boys and girls won't benefit from aerobic and anaerobic training to the same degree as older players, and weight training can be dangerous if not properly supervised. You must also consider that children mature physically at different rates, even within a given age group. This poses additional problems when trying to estimate the appropriate training dosage. The aggregate of these factors leads us to the logical conclusion that specific fitness training is not for kids.

## Fitness Training for Females

Women's soccer is enjoying tremendous popular growth at all levels of competition. Of the 18 million Americans who played soccer last year, more than 7 million were women. The success of our women's national and Olympic teams, coupled with the rapid expansion of women's high school and collegiate soccer, has brought increased exposure to the female side of the sport. Although there has been less research done on the women's game, sport scientists generally agree that females and males require a similar type of fitness to play successfully at a high level. Match analysis indicates that women and men cover a similar distance during a game, and it also appears that a similar proportion of the time is devoted to exercise

> Sport scientists agree that females and males require a similar level of fitness to play successfully at a high level.

of varying intensities. Women, like their male counterparts, require high levels of aerobic fitness, muscular strength and endurance, speed endurance, flexibility and agility to cope with the demands of high level competition.

## Principles Of Fitness Training

### 1. READINESS

To derive the greatest benefit you must be physically and mentally prepared to train hard on a regular basis. This is referred to as your "state of readiness." An individual's state of readiness is influenced by factors such as physical maturity, adequate nutrition and rest, and psychological preparedness. You must be in an optimal state of readiness in order to train on a consistent basis at a high level of intensity. As stated earlier, there are no shortcuts to success.

### 2. RESPONSE TO TRAINING

No two players will respond to training in exactly the same manner. This phenomenon is due to several factors, a few of which are discussed here.

*Maturity*

Maturity is related to an individual's state of readiness. Younger, physically immature players are not capable of handling the same work load as older, more physically developed individuals. In addition, younger players often lack the mental discipline needed to commit to a training program. Lack of physical and mental maturity is one important reason why fitness training should not be a prime concern with pre-adolescent children.

*Initial Level of Fitness*

The lower your initial state of fitness, the more quickly you will see positive results. As your level of fitness improves, however, it will require more intense training to generate continued physical improvement.

*Adaptation to Physical Stress*

The human body is quite amazing in the sense that it will gradually adapt to the physical stress imposed upon it. That is how fitness training works! Your body slowly adjusts (becomes more fit) to handle the increased work load. The physical changes that result in response to training occur on a subtle but consistent basis. For this reason you must progress slowly. You can't get inshape overnight.

*Nutrition and Rest*

Improvements in your overall level of fitness are due in part to changes that occur on a cellular basis. Without sufficient rest and proper nutrition these changes won't occur, and the potential gains derived from fitness training will be minimized.

*Heredity*

We inherit a number of attributes that place limits on our potential for physical development. Muscle fiber characteristics, skeletal type, heart and lung size, and physique are a few such examples. Genetics should never be an excuse for a lack of fitness, however. If we develop to our full potential, whatever that may be, we will be more than ready to excel at the game of soccer.

## 3. OVERLOAD

Fitness activities must place a demand on our physiological systems in order to get the desired results. This concept is often referred to as the training overload. For example, to improve strength you must overload your muscles beyond the point to which they are normally stressed. The same principle applies to your cardiovascular system for aerobic and anaerobic conditioning. As physiological systems gradually adapt to the increased training load, you must then increase the workload even further to stimulate continued progress. The training overload is achieved through manipulation of three variables – frequency, intensity, and time (duration) of exercise. You can easily remember these variables by combining the first letter of each to form the acronym FIT.

> The training overload is achieved through manipulation of three variables – frequency, intensity, and time (duration) of exercise.

## 4. PROGRESSION

Take small steps rather than large leaps when applying the overload principle. Increase the training load in small increments as your body adapts to the physical demands of training. Attempting to do too much too soon will slow your progress, and also increase the likelihood of injury. Increase the workload by making gradual adjustments in the frequency, intensity and/or duration of your training.

## 5. SPECIFICITY

There is a great deal of wisdom in the old coaching adage that says "practice like you play." Adaptations to fitness training are highly specific to the type of activities involved, and to the quantity and intensity of the exercise performed. Training should replicate, as closely as possible, the conditions under which the game is played. Otherwise you won't get the desired results. World class sprinters don't train for the 100 meter dash by running marathons, and soccer players can't adequately prepare for the physiological demands of soccer by simply jogging laps around the field. Training must be specific! It is essential that you set up a schedule and establish training goals. If your goal is to improve speed, then you must train at high speed in practice. To improve general endurance you must overload your aerobic energy systems. To improve strength and power the focus must be on overloading your musculature. The Principle of Specificity is commonly referred to as the S.A.I.D Principle - Specific Adaptations to Imposed Demands.

The S.A.I.D. Principle is closely aligned with our previously stated philosophy of including a ball in your fitness training. For example, you can improve stamina as well as dribbling speed by performing wind sprints while dribbling a ball. Small-sided ( 2 vs. 2, 3 vs. 3) possession games will stress your aerobic and anaerobic systems, and at the same time serve to develop your passing, receiving and dribbling skills. In short, you will benefit from doing as much fitness training with the ball as possible under game-simulated conditions.

### 6. HARD - EASY - HARD TRAINING RHYTHM

With respect to exercise, more is not always better. If you train too long, too hard, and too fast, day after day, week after week, your body will eventually break down and performance will diminish. This condition is often referred to as overtraining or staleness. Muscles need adequate time to recover after a bout of intense training. Physiological adaptations will occur best when fitness training consists of intervals of hard work interspersed with periods of easier work. You can achieve variation in your workouts by using a variety of exercises and by changing your routine.

### 7. LONG HAUL VIEW

A gradual overload of the body's physiological systems leads to the greatest improvements in fitness. Trying to rush the process will only serve to slow down, or even reverse, your progress. The greatest improvements in fitness come to those who commit to a program for the long haul. Fitness must be a year-round endeavor.

### 8. REVERSIBILITY

Just as your fitness will improve through participation in a properly designed training regimen, you can just as easily get out of shape once you stop training. In fact, it takes far less time to get out of shape than it does to get in shape. Sport scientists refer to this phenomenon as the principle of reversibility. Reversibility occurs very quickly for aerobic endurance. If we fail to stress our aerobic energy systems on a regular basis we lose some of our ability to use oxygen efficiently. Reversibility sets in at a much slower pace for muscular strength and power, and is usually the result of atrophy to the muscles. The only way to avoid reversibility is to maintain a year-round fitness program. As the saying goes, "use it or lose it."

## Warm-up and Cool-Down

Always warm up before each practice and game so as to physically and mentally prepare yourself for high intensity activity. Warm-up exercises fulfill several important functions. Muscle temperatures become elevated which promotes increased blood flow. This in turn allows for improved muscle contraction and reflex time, increased suppleness, and helps to prevent next-day soreness. A thorough warm-up also guards against muscle, tendon, and ligament injuries. The length and intensity of warm-up can vary depending upon individual needs and the surrounding environmental conditions (temperature, humidity, etc.). Obviously you won't have to work as hard to warm your muscles on a sunny, humid day in July as you might on a cold, windy day in November. As a rule of thumb, warm up for 15 to 20 minutes at sufficient intensity to cause sweating. Perspiration is an indication that your muscle temperatures have been elevated.

Any activity that involves large muscle groups can be used in the warm-up. A traditional warm-up consists of stretching exercises and calisthenics like jumping jacks, sit-ups, toe-raises, and push-ups. This type of warm-up is commonly referred to as an "unrelated" warm-up because it does not involve sport-specific movements. From a practical standpoint, it is better to undergo a "related" warm-up composed of soccer-specific movements

> The greatest improvements in fitness come to those who commit to program for the long haul. Fitness must be a year-round endeavor.

and activities. This could include a variety of skill-related drills that involve passing, receiving, or dribbling a soccer ball. Goalkeepers can use various types of foot movements and ball handling activities, as well as flexibility and agility exercises. Both related and unrelated warm-ups can achieve the desired physiological changes. When possible, however, use a related warm-up because you also get the benefit of a practice effect.

A cool-down period at the end of practice is just as important as the warm-up prior to training. The cool-down is designed to slowly bring your body back to its normal state of homeostasis. For example, a light jog with the ball after completion of a hard training session gradually lowers your heart rate to within normal limits, and also helps to maintain the pumping action of muscles on veins which aids in the removal of metabolic wastes. During the cool-down you should select a static stretch exercise for each major muscle group and thoroughly stretch that area. Include the hamstrings and quadriceps, groin, and lower back. Stretching during the cool-down will help prevent next-day soreness and also allows your body temperature to gradually return to normal.

## Treatment of Injuries

Try as you might to avoid them, injuries will undoubtedly occur at some point during the practice or playing season. Because a critical element of fitness training is simply the ability to train on a consistent basis, it is important that you know how to treat injuries to ensure the swiftest possible recovery.

Most soccer injuries occur below the waist. The three most common injuries are sprains, strains and contusions. A sprain is an injury to a ligament. Ligaments are the connective tissue bands that attach bones to bones, such as the ligaments that stabilize your knee. A strain is an injury to a muscle or tendon. Tendons are the connective tissues that attach muscles to bones. Contusions are bruises to muscles or soft tissue where bleeding occurs. All three of these injuries should be treated using the R.I.C.E. Principle. R.I.C.E. is the acronym for **rest, ice, compression,** and **elevation,** and is the recommended treatment during the first 24 to 48 hours following an injury. The standard procedure is as follows. The injured player should be removed from the practice or game. This is the *rest* phase of treatment. *Ice* is immediately applied to the injured area in a crushed ice bag or chemical pack, preferably with a damp cloth placed between the skin and ice to prevent tissue damage. *Compression* is then applied through the use of

# SAMPLE WARM-UP

5 minutes: Light jogging while:
1. dribbling a ball while changing speed and direction
2. juggling a ball with feet and thighs
3. juggling a ball with head

5 minutes: Flexibility exercises (static stretches)
Agility/footwork exercises

10-15 minutes: Group warm-up activities with the ball (5 minutes each)

## 1. Numbers Passing Game

Use markers to outline a 30 by 40 yard area. Play with a group of six teammates. Number each player in the group, beginning with #1 and ending with #6. Two players each have possession of a ball to begin. All players begin jogging within the area; the two with a ball dribble it. Those players with a ball locate the teammate numbered directly above and pass to him or her. Player #6 passes to player #1 to complete the circuit. All players move continuously throughout the exercise as they pass to the teammate numbered above them and receive passes from the teammate numbered below them (the number of players can vary).

## 2. Shadow Dribble

Pair with a partner. Each of you has a ball. Your partner begins to dribble randomly throughout the field area, while you closely follow .Your goal is to imitate, or shadow, the movements and dribbling maneuvers of your partner. Change positions every 60 seconds; you become the leader and your partner follows.

## 3. Takeover Drill

Join with 8 to 10 teammates. Every other player has possession of a ball to begin. All players begin moving randomly throughout a 30 yard square field area. Those with a ball dribble, those without a ball jog at half-speed. At their discretion the dribblers exchange possession of their ball with one of the free players, using the proper takeover technique. As they prepare to exchange possession the dribblers should control the ball with the foot farthest from an imaginary defender.

an ace bandage, or possibly a towel secured with elastic bands. Finally, the injured area should be *elevated* above heart level to slow the blood flow. It is important that the R.I.C.E. treatment begin immediately after an injury has occurred. As a general rule, the longer the delay the longer the recovery time.

## Common Training Myths

It is often difficult and confusing to separate fact from fiction when it comes to fitness training. Everyone has a different philosophy of "what works." The following material discusses a few commonly held beliefs about fitness and exercise that are, in fact, false.

### 1. "NO PAIN, NO GAIN" – IT'S GOT TO HURT TO BE WORTHWHILE...

The "go for the burn" mentality has been perpetuated by a minority of misguided coaches, trainers, and athletes. Granted, exercise intensity is an important factor when trying to attain a high level of fitness. However, you don't have to train so hard that it hurts in order to get results. You will obviously experience some discomfort as you progressively overload your systems, and that is to be expected. Discomfort is a natural consequence of stressing the muscles or cardiovascular system. Intense pain, however, is a different story. Pain is a warning signal that says "ease up." Slow and steady improvement wins the fitness race.

### 2. THE MORE I SWEAT THE MORE FAT I WILL LOSE...

This school of thought spawned the popularity of vinyl or rubber exercise suits designed to "sweat it off." You should absolutely not wear these types of suits! The extra weight that you lose when working out in a rubber suit is due to fluid loss, not fat loss. Not only do such suits fail to promote increased fat loss, but they may also cause serious health problems. The rubber or vinyl fabric prevents your body from effectively using its built-in cooling system, sweat. Dehydration and heat stroke can occur.

### 3. UNEXERCISED MUSCLES WILL TURN INTO FAT...

This belief is based upon a perception of the young, muscular athlete gradually changing into a pudgy, middle-aged ex-jock once the playing days have ended. To the casual observer it appears that muscle has turned into fat. In truth, muscles cells and fat cells are entirely distinct tissues. One cannot change into the other. It is true that muscles will atrophy, become smaller, and lose strength due to a lack of exercise. The deposition of body fat, however, is purely and simply the result of taking in more energy (calories) than is needed to fuel daily activities. Over a period of time the combination of muscle atrophy and fat deposition can give the impression that muscle has somehow been transformed into fat, but that is not actually the case.

### 4. TO GAIN MUSCLE I MUST EAT MORE PROTEIN...

The benefits of protein supplements have been greatly exaggerated. While it is true that protein plays an important role in the growth and repair of cells, eating excessive amounts of protein will not transform small, soft muscles into huge, well defined muscles. Only strength training will do that. Eating too much protein may actually be detrimental because its breakdown places added strain on the liver and kidneys. If you are presently eating a normal American diet, then you are probably getting more than enough protein to satisfy any increased needs due to exercise.

### 5. LIFTING WEIGHTS WILL MAKE ME MUSCLE-BOUND...

The fear of getting muscle-bound and losing flexibility has discouraged many soccer players from lifting weights. In truth, a properly supervised weight program designed specifically to improve soccer performance can only make you a better athlete. Resistance training will improve your muscular strength, endurance and power, and also lessens the likelihood of muscular injury. It is important to use proper lifting technique, perform each exercise through a full range of motion, and stretch after every strength training session.

## Summary

Many factors interact to determine a soccer player's level of performance. Technical ability, tactical knowledge, psychological preparation, and level of fitness each play a role. All other things being equal, however, the player who is more physically fit will generally achieve a higher standard of performance on the playing field. Important elements of soccer-related fitness include aerobic and anaerobic capacity, flexibility, agility, muscular strength, muscular endurance, and power. The exercises and activities used to develop fitness should center around these parameters, and should simulate as closely as possible the movements and physiological demands encountered during a game.

# 3 Aerobic Fitness

Endurance is a general term that actually refers to two distinct yet related fitness components: cardiorespiratory and muscular endurance. The degree to which each plays a role in athletic performance depends upon the physiological demands of the sport in question. For example, a sprinter who runs the 100 meter dash requires a specific type of fitness to maintain maximum speed over the full distance.

In this case we are talking about muscular endurance - the ability of a single muscle or muscle group to sustain high-intensity, repetitive exercise. Muscular endurance is very important in sports that require repetitive, explosive movements of relatively short duration. Cardiorespiratory endurance, also called aerobic fitness, deals with the body as a whole rather than with specific muscles. In a technical sense, aerobic fitness can be defined as the maximal capacity to take in, transport, and utilize oxygen. It is a measure of your ability to sustain prolonged, sub-maximal activity, and is determined in large part by the ability of your circulatory system to provide sufficient oxygen to the working muscles.

Soccer players must develop high levels of both aerobic and muscular endurance. An aerobic fitness base enables you to sustain a high level of sub-maximal continuous effort for the entire 90 minutes of a match. Muscular endurance enables you to perform the high intensity explosive-type movements frequently observed during a game. These include sprinting runs, kicking and jumping movements, explosive bursts of speed, and sudden changes of direction. The fundamental aspects of aerobic fitness are discussed here. Muscular endurance, an essential component of muscular fitness, is covered in Chapter 5.

## Aerobic Capacity

The word aerobic literally means "in the presence of oxygen." The energy used for aerobic activity comes from the oxidation of fat and carbohydrates. During aerobic exercise you are taking in sufficient oxygen to supply the active tissues' immediate needs. Once the intensity of exercise goes beyond your ability to supply sufficient oxygen to the muscles, the body automatically shifts to anaerobic (without oxygen) energy production. Anaerobic activities generally involve maximum effort of short duration. During anaerobic energy production lactic acid accumulates in the muscles and blood, a signal that you are using energy faster than you can produce it aerobically. Lactic acid is both an energy transporter and a by-product of intense effort. Excessive build-up of lactic acid interferes with muscle function and metabolic activities, and causes feelings of fatigue and discomfort. That is one of the primary reasons why you can't remain in an anaerobic state for extended periods of time – it doesn't feel very good! Aerobic activity is performed at intensities below the level at which blood lactate acid levels rise rapidly, a point that is commonly referred to as the lactate threshold. Soccer players fluctuate between aerobic and anaerobic energy states throughout the course of a game.

The transport and delivery of oxygen to the working muscles during aerobic

> Soccer players must develop high levels of both aerobic and muscular endurance.

exercise is carried out by your cardiovascular and respiratory systems. Components of these two systems that are related to oxygen transport are collectively referred to as the "oxygen transport system." Endurance training elicits positive changes in the oxygen transport system enabling it to function more efficiently. This, in turn, increases your ability to perform sustained, high

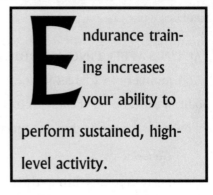

Endurance training increases your ability to perform sustained, high-level activity.

level activity. You are able to exercise harder for longer periods of time without reaching the lactate threshold.

Sport scientists generally regard VO2 max as the best measure of aerobic power. VO2 max, measured in milliliters per kilogram of body weight per minute (ml/kg/min), is defined as the highest rate of oxygen consumption attainable during exhaustive exercise. The higher your VO2 max, the greater aerobic workload you can sustain. Oxygen consumption will either plateau or even decrease slightly as exercise intensity goes beyond the point of VO2 max. In this physiological state your oxygen transport system is unable to supply the tissues with sufficient oxygen, a condition commonly referred to as oxygen debt. You cannot sustain exercise for very long in a state of oxygen debt, and performance soon diminishes. From that perspective you can understand how a high level of aerobic endurance is your best defense against fatigue.

Physical and mental fatigue pose an obstacle to optimal performance for endurance athletes, and can be particularly detrimental to soccer players who must execute highly skilled movements throughout 90 minutes of intense physical stress. Fatigue due to an inadequate level of aerobic fitness has the following effects:

√ reduces muscular strength

√ slows reaction times

√ slows whole-body movement

√ impairs agility and coordination

√ lessens mental alertness and the ability to concentrate

All of these factors impact soccer performance. Even a slight reduction in one or more of the above will have a detrimental effect on your ability to compete at a high level.

## FACTORS AFFECTING AEROBIC FITNESS

A number of variables interact to determine your level of aerobic fitness at any point in time. Some of these factors are within your control, and some are not. The following is a brief discussion of factors affecting aerobic fitness.

### Genetics

There is some truth to the statement that "great athletes are born, not made." We do inherit certain characteristics that contribute to determining our maximal aerobic capacity. These factors include the size of our heart, the maximal capacity of our respiratory system, the density of red cells and hemoglobin, and the percentage of slow-twitch and fast-twitch muscle fibers. We also inherit mitochondria, the energy-producing units of muscles and other cells. At first glance these findings appear to lead to the logical conclusion that, if you expect to play soccer at a high level, you had better choose your parents carefully! Thankfully, that conclusion is not totally correct. Regardless of our short-comings, we still possess the ability to determine our athletic destiny. Determination, persistence, and proper training are the keys to achieving our goals.

### Gender

Prior to puberty there is little difference between boys and girls in aerobic fitness. As we get older, however, girls begin to lag behind. Young women average 15 to 25% less aerobic capacity than young men. It appears that this difference is, at least in part, due to differing activity levels. Although times are changing, women as a group are still not as physically active as men. Activity levels can't account for all of the difference however. Studies show that even highly trained female endurance athletes generally score lower in VO2 max than men of similar age. One reason may be the fact that men average more hemoglobin, the oxygen-carrying compound found in red blood cells, than do women. Total hemoglobin is highly correlated with endurance capacity. Women also average more body fat than men, are generally smaller, and have less muscle mass, all factors that tend to limit aerobic endurance. Even so, the tremendous improvements demonstrated by women over the past decade in events like the marathon run clearly show that females can develop high levels of aerobic fitness if provided the same training opportunities as males.

*Percent Body Fat*

Because aerobic fitness (VO2 Max) is calculated per unit of body weight, your level of fitness automatically declines as you get fatter. Carrying excess fat also limits your mobility and agility. Proven methods used to achieve optimal weight are discussed in detail in Chapter 11.

*Training*

Although genetics may place a limit on our aerobic potential, few of us ever actually reach that upper boundary. The vast majority of soccer players can improve their level of aerobic fitness, at least to a limited extent, through proper training. Aerobic conditioning improves the efficiency of our oxygen transport system by increasing blood volume and oxygen carrying capacity. Important adaptations also occur in the muscle fibers specifically used in aerobic training. The muscles' ability to produce energy aerobically improves as metabolism is shifted from carbohydrate to fat. The primary aims of aerobic fitness training for soccer players are the following:

1. To improve the ability of the cardiovascular and respiratory systems to transport oxygen. This will enable a larger amount of the energy to be supplied aerobically, which in turn allows you to perform at higher exercise intensity for a longer period of time.

2. To improve the muscles' capacity to utilize oxygen and to oxidize fat during prolonged periods of activity. This allows your body to spare its limited stores of muscle glycogen for use during the later stages of a game when it is really needed.

3. To improve your ability to recover quickly after a bout of high-

intensity exercise. This is a particularly important aspect for soccer players because the rhythm and intensity of play is constantly changing.

## Components of Aerobic Training

Aerobic fitness training can be divided into three overlapping components.

### LOW INTENSITY AEROBIC TRAINING

Your endurance capacity can be improved through continuous or intermittent activity of sufficient intensity to maintain heart rate within a training zone of 60 to 80% of maximum. This type of low- to medium-intensity training is often called LSD - long, slow distance. Quantity (distance) of exercise is emphasized over quality (speed). Heart rate seldom gets above 160 beats per minute during the activity.

Low intensity aerobic training can be accomplished through a variety of soccer-related drills and small-sided game competitions. Distance running and fartlek can be used when training without a ball. Fartlek, or speed play, was developed in Sweden during the 1930's. Initially used to train distance runners, fartlek is a form of continuous training performed in an internal fashion. A fartlek run may last 45 minutes or more and cover several miles. The pace fluctuates between periods of high intensity sprinting and slow jogging. Fartlek is usually performed over varied terrain as opposed to a flat track.

### HIGH INTENSITY AEROBIC TRAINING

Studies show that the amount of high intensity running during a game is related to the level of competition. As one would expect, the top players cover the most ground at the highest intensities. So, if your goal is to play at a highly competitive level, you must be physically able to accept that challenge. High intensity aerobic training is performed at intensities that represent 85 to 95% of an athlete's maximal heart rate. In addition to improving cardiovascular endurance, high intensity aerobic training also develops leg strength, leg speed, and muscular endurance.

### RECOVERY TRAINING

You need not and actually should not train hard every day. The day after a game, or possibly the day after a high intensity training session, are good times to lighten the training load to allow your body time to recuperate. Recovery training usually consists of low intensity exercises with the ball. Activities can include dribbling, passing, shooting, and possession games performed at sub-maximal effort. Low intensity "fun" game competitions are also an effective means of breaking a sweat while enjoying some lighthearted fun. During recovery training your mean heart rate should center around 130 beats per minute.

## Planning Your Program

Take into account four factors — frequency, duration, intensity, and mode — when planning the aerobic portion of your comprehensive fitness program. Mode refers to the type of activity which, for soccer players, should replicate the game as much as possible. Frequency, duration, and intensity are more concerned with the quality and quantity of exercise. You must exceed a minimum threshold for each of these factors to realize a training effect. Training thresholds vary from one person to another, however, depending upon initial level of fitness. For example, an individual who is very fit to begin with will have to train at a greater intensity (higher threshold) than the player whose

> In addition to improving cardio-vascular endurance, high intensity aerobic training also develops leg strength, leg speed, and muscular endurance.

initial level of fitness is very low in order to get a similar training effect. Individual differences in response to aerobic exercise must also be taken into account. The bottom line is that there isn't one magical formula that works best for everyone. You must experiment to find out what works best for you.

### FREQUENCY

Soccer players must train aerobically a minimum of five days per week, and preferably more frequently, to achieve a high level of aerobic fitness. If your fitness level is low to begin with due to an extended period of inactivity, three sessions per week on alternating days is probably enough to generate initial fitness gains. As fitness improves, however, the frequency of training must also increase in order to stimulate continued progress. Follow the hard-easy principle — long bouts of high intensity training should be followed by shorter bouts of less intense training. Failure to allow adequate recovery can diminish the positive effects of high intensity fitness training, and may eventually result in overuse injuries and staleness.

As fitness improves, the frequency of training must also increase in order to stimulate continued progress.

### DURATION

The volume of training is usually measured in time, distance, or both. The average non-athlete individual can realize positive health benefits with as little as twenty minutes per session three times per week. Soccer players must train more frequently and for longer duration, however, to significantly improve stamina and performance. Research suggests that similar fitness benefits can result from both a shorter duration high intensity program and a longer-duration lower intensity program. The key ingredient appears to be matching the optimal threshold for duration with appropriate exercise intensity.

### INTENSITY

Exercise intensity is the most critical factor affecting improvements in aerobic capacity. It reflects the amount of oxygen consumed, the energy requirements of the exercise, and the energy expended. Heart rate is the most commonly used measure of exercise intensity because it is highly correlated with the amount of  work being performed. Aerobic fitness training must exceed a minimum level of intensity, or *threshold*, in order for physiological adaptations to occur. The minimum training threshold, referred to as the aerobic threshold, will vary among individuals depending upon their initial level of fitness. The higher your initial fitness level the harder you must work to generate improvements in fitness. There is also an upper threshold for aerobic training beyond which the contribution to aerobic fitness diminishes. This upper limit coincides with the anaerobic (lactate) threshold. Training at intensities above the lactate threshold will not contribute significantly to the development of aerobic fitness, but it does provide other fitness benefits. Anaerobic training and its effects are discussed in the Chapter 4.

## Determining Your Training Zone

The minimum intensity threshold needed to improve cardiovascular fitness is approximately 60% of your maximum heart rate (MHR), the maximum number of times your heart can beat in a minute. You can estimate MHR by subtracting your age in years from 220. For example, a 20 year old soccer player would have an approximate MHR of 200 beats per minute (bpm). It is best to establish a heart rate range, or zone, rather than a single value to allow for progressive increases in exercise intensity. The training heart rate zone for aerobic fitness ranges between 60 and 90 percent of your MHR. Multiply MHR by 0.6 to get the lower threshold of the target training zone. Multiply by 0.9 to get the upper limit. A 20-year old player would have a lower threshold of 120 bpm and an upper limit of 180 bpm.

It is relatively easy to monitor heart rate during exercise. Stop exercising for a moment and locate your pulse by resting the index and middle finger at the base of your wrist, or at the side of your neck near your Adam's apple. Count the heart beats for 15 seconds and multiply by four to get your heart rate. That number should be somewhere between the lower and upper boundaries of your training zone. After a while you will be able to judge whether you are in the "zone" simply by listening to what your body tells you. Cues such as sweating, breathing patterns, and aching muscles help you to gauge exercise intensity. Keep in mind that, as your fitness level improves, your heart rate will decrease for the same amount of work. In other words, as you become fitter you will have to work harder to reach your training threshold.

## Training for the Game

Always keep in mind that you must not only train to be fit, but also must also train to be a soccer player! Physiological adaptations that occur in response to aerobic training are highly specific to the type, volume and intensity of the activity. Common sense dictates that you structure your training around the movements, muscles, metabolic pathways, and support systems used in soccer. In other words, train for the demands of the match! The following games can be used towards that aim. Each is designed to improve fitness as well as technical ability with the ball. You can manipulate variables within each game (i.e., the number of touches of the ball allowed, size of the area, duration of the activity, etc.) to make the training more or less demanding.

**SOCCER-RELATED GAMES TO DEVELOP AEROBIC FITNESS**

1. **Slalom Dribble.** Place 8 markers in single file with 3 yards distance between cones. Beginning at the first marker, dribble as fast as possible through the slalom course, weaving in and out of the markers front to back to front. Complete three complete circuits of the course, rest for an equal amount of time, and then repeat. The work:rest ratio is 1:1.

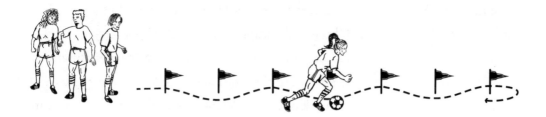

2. **Keep Away.** Play keep away against a teammate in a 15 by 20 yard area. You begin with possession of the ball, your teammate plays as the defender. Use sudden changes of speed and direction coupled with dribbling maneuvers to keep the ball from the defender. Play for 30 seconds, rest for 30 seconds, and repeat. Play 10 rounds as an attacker, then switch roles and play 10 rounds as the defender. The work:rest ratio is 1:1.

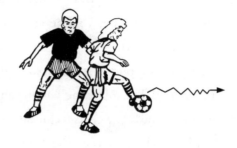

#3 . **One-versus-one to a Central Goal.** Pair with a partner. Use markers to outline a field area 20 yards square; place a pair of cones to represent a common goal 1 yard wide in the center of the area. Play one-versus-one within the area. Goals can be scored from either side of the central goal. Change of possession occurs when your opponent steals the ball or when the ball travels outside of the field area. Play a series of 1-minute games with a rest of 60 seconds between games. The work:rest ratio is 1:1.

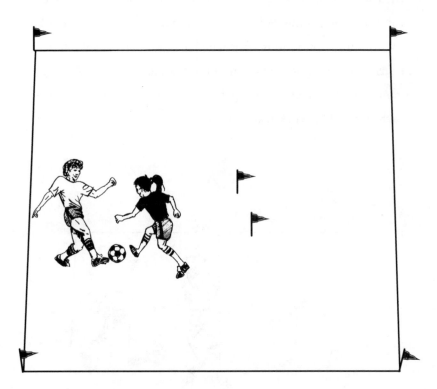

4. **One-versus-one with Support.** Form two teams of two players each. Use markers to outline a 15 by 25 yard field. One player on each team positions as a goal by standing with feet spread apart on his or her respective end line. The remaining players compete one-versus-one in the center of the area. The player with the ball scores by dribbling past his or her opponent and passing the ball through the legs of the "goal". Players positioned as goals must remain stationary and cannot stop the ball from rolling through their legs. Change of possession occurs when the defender steals the ball, or when the ball travels out of play, or after a score. Play two-minutes continuous after which central players switch positions with their goalkeeper and play resumes. Play ten 2-minute games, with players rotating between the field and goal after each game. The work:rest ratio is 1:1.

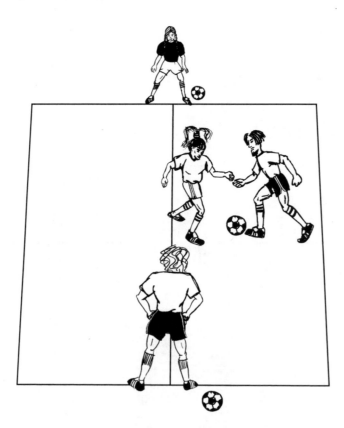

5. **Possession Game.** Form two teams of three players each. Use markers to outline a playing area of 25 yards square. Award one team possession of the ball to begin. The team with the ball (attacking team) attempts to keep it from the defending team through combination interpassing and/or dribbling skills. Change of possession occurs when the defending team steals the ball, or when the ball travels outside of the field area. Team roles reverse immediately upon change of possession. The attacking team is awarded 1 point for 6 consecutive passes without loss of possession. Play continuously for 20 minutes; the team scoring the most points wins the game.

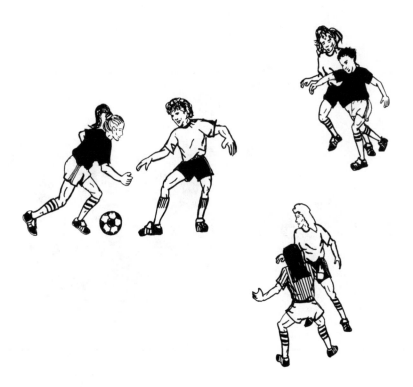

6. **One-on-One Marking Game.** Form two teams of five players each. Use markers to outline a playing field 30 by 40 yards with a goal 3 yards wide positioned at the center of each end line. Each team defends a goal; do not use goalkeepers. Require strict one-versus-one marking of opponents. Shots may be taken from any distance so marking must be very tight to prevent long-range scores. The one-versus-one marking restriction increases the fitness demands of the exercise because defending players are forced to apply pressure on opponents all over the field. The team scoring the most goals wins the game. Play continuously for 25 minutes.

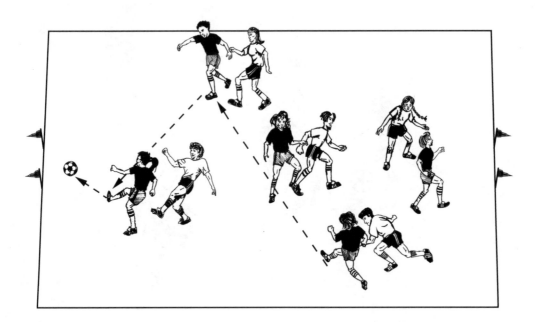

7. **Score Through Back Door or Front Door.** Organize teams of two or three players each. Use markers to outline a 35 yard square. Position cones or flags to represent two small goals within the playing area. Do not use goalkeepers; award one team possession of the ball to begin. Regular soccer rules apply except that teams can score by kicking the ball through either goal. In addition, goals may be scored from both sides of the goals, providing the opportunity to score through the "front door" or the "back door". Play for 20 minutes.

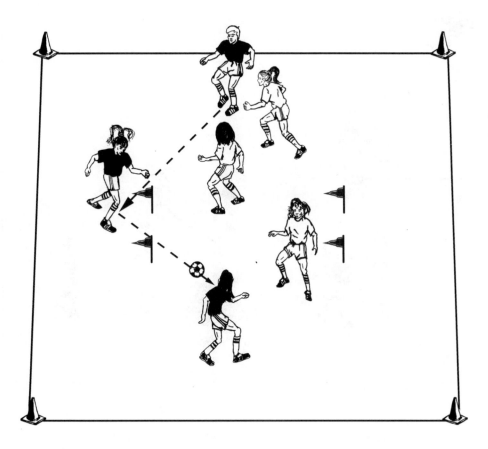

8. **Score by Dribbling Only.** Organize teams of 4 to 6 players each. Play on a 40 by 65 yard field area. Award one team possession of the ball to begin. Each team defends an end line of the field. Regular soccer rules apply, except that goals are scored by dribbling the ball over an opponents' end line rather than by shooting the ball into a goal. Require one-versus-one marking to increase the physical demands of the game. Play for 30 minutes.

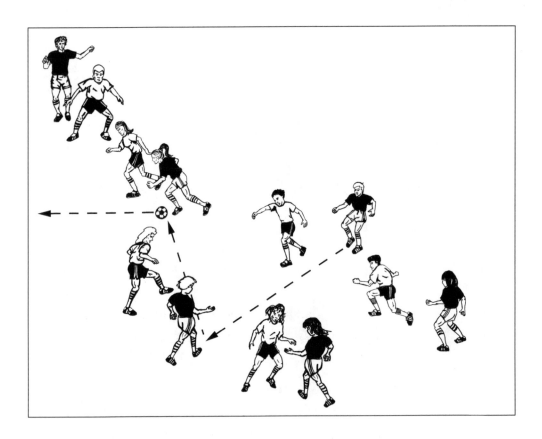

# 4 Anaerobic Fitness

Although much of the activity during a soccer game is at sub-maximal intensity, you must also train your muscles and energy systems for the frequent bouts of high intensity effort that occur intermittently throughout a match. The aerobic training discussed in Chapter 3 consisted of sub-maximal exercise, or activity below the lactate (VO2) threshold. Anaerobic training deals with exercise intensities above the lactate threshold. Obviously, at times, there will be overlap of anaerobic and aerobic training since exercise intensity will vary within a game or specific fitness activity.

In general, however, anaerobic training is of shorter duration and higher intensity than aerobic training. For that reason aerobic training is commonly referred to as quantity, or volume, training while anaerobic training is considered to be quality training. The difference between aerobic and anaerobic training is not so much what you do, but rather how hard you do it. Anaerobic activities require near-maximal force production. Exercise at 90 to 100% of maximum heart rate guarantees that the work is anaerobic. The objectives of anaerobic training for soccer players are:

1. To improve your ability to respond instantly and produce power rapidly during high-intensity exercise. For example, the ability to suddenly change direction and explode past a defender can be improved through anaerobic training.

2. To improve your capacity to produce power and energy via the anaerobic energy-producing pathways. This will enable you to perform higher-intensity activity for a longer period of time during a game.

3. To decrease the time required to recover after a period of high intensity effort. The more quickly you can recover from a bout of maximal effort, the sooner you can do it again.

## Methods of Anaerobic Training

Anaerobic training is generally divided into two related categories: speed training and speed endurance training. The objective of speed training is to improve your absolute running speed, while speed endurance training develops your ability to maintain maximal speed for a longer period of time.

### SPEED TRAINING

The potential for running at speed is, for the most part, genetically determined. If you were born with a preponderance of slow twitch (endurance) rather than fast twitch (explosive movement) muscle fiber, then you will never be an Olympic sprint champion. That does not mean, however, that you can't improve your running speed. Through intense anaerobic training and efficient running form you can increase, to a limited extent, your absolute sprinting speed.

Soccer players will benefit from two forms of speed training. Acceleration sprints are characterized by a gradual increase in speed until reaching maximum sprint speed. Start the run by jogging, gradually increase your stride and speed, and end up sprinting the final leg. For example, if you are sprinting cross field from one touchline to the other, you would jog the first 15 yards, stride the next 20 yards, and cover the final 30 to 40 yards at maximum speed. Active recovery between acceleration sprints, such as slowly jogging or walking back to the starting line, is recommended. Acceleration sprints are an effective means of improving running speed because you can focus on your technique and stride length during the build-up phase of the sprint. They also minimize the likelihood of muscle pulls and strains because you gradually build to full-sprint speed.

The second type of speed training is aptly called sprint training. When sprint training the entire run, from beginning to end, is performed at maximum speed. The rest interval between sprints should be sufficient to allow near-complete recovery. Sprint training is considered to be high quality, maximum effort anaerobic training.

The potential for running at speed is, for the most part, genetically determined.

### SPEED ENDURANCE TRAINING

Speed endurance training is designed to improve your ability to perform high-intensity running repeatedly during a game. It involves training of the anaerobic (lactate-producing) energy pathways, and can be accomplished through fartlek training at high intensities, or better yet, through high intensity games. The muscular adaptations resulting from speed endurance training are specific to the exercising muscles, so it is important that players perform movements similar to those used in match play. This can be accomplished through high intensity drills that involve a ball. (See Figure 4.1.)

## The Interval Training Format

Research has demonstrated that athletes can perform considerably more work if they break the work into short, intense bouts with periods of rest between consecutive bouts. This is commonly referred to as the interval method of training. The interval format can be adapted to virtually any endurance-type sport, and is particularly applicable to soccer fitness training.

Interval training can be effectively used to develop both anaerobic and aerobic endurance. As the term "interval' implies, exercise alternates between periods of intense physical effort (work) followed by periods of recovery (rest). The rhythm of

### Figure 4.1 Breakaway and Score Drill

**Objective:** Speed endurance training, development of dribbling speed.

**Area of Field:** Play on one-half of a regulation field with a regulation size goal on the end line.

**Number of Players:** Groups of two; three to five groups.

**Organization:** Players work in pairs. Two players jog randomly within the center circle. A server kicks a ball toward goal. Both players immediately leave the circle and sprint to the ball. The player reaching the ball first becomes the attacker and tries to score; the other player becomes the defender. Players compete at maximum effort until the attacker scores a goal or defender kicks the ball away. Players rest while next pair plays. The work:rest interval should be approximately 1:3 or 1:4.

**Practice Tips:** Player gaining control of the ball should be encouraged to make a direct run to goal and shoot.

interval training (hard-easy-hard) closely simulates the type of physical stress encountered in a match. An added advantage of interval training is its flexible format – the program can be adapted to meet individual needs and abilities. The intensity of a workout can be manipulated simply by adjusting variables in the work schedule. These variables include:

√ intensity of effort during the work interval

√ length of time of work interval

√ number of repetitions of work interval

√ length (time) of rest interval

√ activity (if any) during rest interval

A variety of fitness drills can be designed using an interval format. The ratio of work to rest, referred to as the "work:rest ratio," can vary depending upon the length of the work interval. The usual ratio is 1:2 or 1:3. This means that the rest interval is either twice as long or three times as long as the work interval. For example, if the drill requires you to dribble a ball back and forth between two lines at maximum speed for 30 seconds (work interval), then the rest interval would be 60 to 90 seconds. As a general rule of thumb, the more fit the athlete the shorter the rest period.

## Adaptations to Anaerobic Training

We've discussed how anaerobic training can improve your ability to sustain high intensity activity for extended periods of time. Anaerobic training can also enhance your soccer performance in other ways as well.

### EFFICIENCY OF MOVEMENT

Training at higher intensities and maximal speeds improves your coordination and ability to execute skills at higher speeds. Training under anaerobic conditions improves muscular efficiency, and enables your muscles to conserve energy that might otherwise be wasted on needless movement.

### AEROBIC BENEFITS

Some forms of anaerobic training also stress the aerobic energy systems. For example, some of the energy used during longer sprints is derived from oxidative metabolism. As a consequence, repeated bouts of sprint-type fitness activity will also increase the muscles' aerobic capacity.

### BUFFERING EFFECT

Anaerobic training improves the muscles' ability to tolerate the lactic acid that accumulates during maximal exercise. This enables sprint-trained athletes to accumulate greater amounts of lactate in their blood and muscles during and following a maximal sprint to exhaustion. In practical terms, an improved ability to tolerate lactic acid delays the onset of fatigue

## Skill Improvement vs. Fitness Training – The Tradeoff

One of the messages I've tried to emphasize throughout the book is that you should, whenever possible, include a ball in your fitness training. Training with a ball enables you to develop two additional performance factors - technical and tactical ability - while also improving your fitness. That being said, sometimes it is difficult to effectively integrate skill or tactical training into a fitness workout without diminishing the fitness aspect of the training. For example, by including a ball in a speed training workout you may improve your ability to dribble at speed, but may also limit improvements in your absolute sprinting speed without the ball. In such cases you must make a choice – do you want to focus on dribbling speed (skill) or absolute running speed (fitness) ? You can't always maximize the training effect for both in the same drill. In some cases each aspect of performance must be addressed separately to realize maximum benefits. Speed training, for the most part, is one of these situations.

In summary, it is difficult to quantify the percentage of a match that is played in an anaerobic state because exercise intensity is constantly changing. It is safe to say, however, that you are in an aerobic state for a greater amount of time during a game than an anaerobic state. As a consequence the energy production from anaerobic metabolism is somewhat less than the energy yield from aerobic metabolism. Nevertheless, development of your anaerobic system is critical to peak soccer performance because it is associated with the high intensity exercise periods that occur during a match.

## Anaerobic Fitness Exercises (with the ball)

To derive anaerobic fitness benefits from the following exercises you must exercise at an effort level between 80 and 90 percent of your maximum heart rate.

1. **Cone to Cone.** Place 2 cones 15 yards apart. Dribble from cone to cone at maximum speed and effort for 30 seconds. Rest 60 seconds, and repeat. The work:rest ratio is 1:2.

2. **Check to the Line.** Stand on the touchline facing a teammate (server) positioned 20 yards away. The server passes a rolling ball toward you. Sprint to the ball, execute a one-touch pass back to the server, turn, and sprint back to the touchline. Continue at maximum speed for 45 seconds, then switch roles with server. The work:rest ratio is 1:1.

3. **Round the Post and Back.** Place two cones 30 yards apart. Position at a cone with a ball. Dribble as fast as possible around the opposite cone and back to the starting point. Rest for twice as long as it took you to complete the circuit, then repeat. Run a total of 6 to 10 sprints with the ball. The work:rest ratio is 1:2

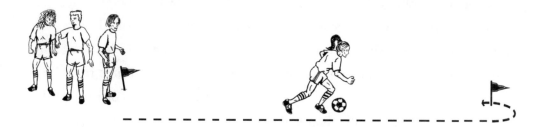

Round the Post and Back drill

4. **Sprint to Goal-Kick.** Goalkeeper stands in goal, one field player positions at each goal post. The keeper kicks the ball down the field and the field players immediately sprint to collect the ball. The first player to the ball is awarded 1 point. After each point players jog back to the goal and the game restarts as before. First player to score 10 points wins the game.

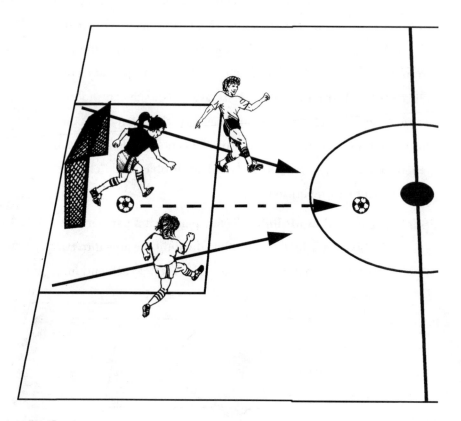

5. **Pass and Follow.** Divide into groups of three. Two players (A & B) position on the goal line; A has possession of the ball. The third player (C) positions on the edge of the penalty area facing A & B. Player A passes the ball to C and immediately sprints to that spot. Player C receives the ball, controls it with his or her first touch, passes to Player B positioned on the goal line, and immediately sprints to that spot. Players A, B and C continue to interchange positions by passing and immediately sprinting to follow their pass. Continue the drill until each player has completed 20 sprints.

6. **Pair Sprinting with Ball.** Play on a normal size field. Pair with a partner within the center circle of the field; one ball required per pair. One player dribbles within the center circle, the other closely follows. At the dribbler's discretion he or she leaves the circle and dribbles as fast as possible towards one of the goals. His or her teammate becomes the defender and attempts to strip the ball from the dribbler before he or she can enter the penalty area. Once the dribbler enters the penalty area he or she can shoot to score. Award the attacker 1 point for a score, the defender 1 point for preventing a score. Players return to center circle after each repetition, and alternate turns playing as dribbler and defender. Perform 10 to 15 repetitions.

7. **Sprinting to Ball at Midline.** Players pair with a partner. Play on a 60 by 40 yard field with a midline dividing the area into two equal halves. Position a small goal at the center of each end line,

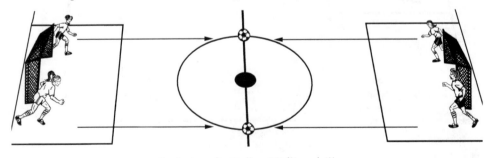

Sprinting the Ball at Midline drill

and a ball on the midline. Partners position on opposite end lines. On the command "go" both players sprint to the ball. Whoever gets there first dribbles toward the goal at the opposite end and attempts to score. The other player defends. Award 1 point for a score. Players return to their respective end line at the end of each repetition. Perform 15 to 20 repetitions.

## Anaerobic Fitness Exercises (without the ball)

8. **Six to Six.** Stand in front of the goal on the six yard line of a regulation-size field. Sprint to the opposite six yard line in 15 or fewer seconds. Rest there for 30 seconds, then sprint back to the original starting point. Run six to eight repetitions of "six to six." Each run must be 15 seconds or less with 30 seconds of rest/recovery between runs. The work:rest ratio is 1:2.

9. **Shuttle Runs.** Place five cones in a straight line with 5 yards distance between cones. Starting at cone #1, sprint to cone #2 and then back to #1, sprint to #3 and back to #1, sprint to #4 and back to #1, sprint to #5, back to #1, and you've finished one repetition. Rest for twice as long as it took you to run the shuttle, then run again. Complete a total of five repetitions of the shuttle.

10. **Union Jacks.** Begin at one corner of a regulation-size field. Sprint diagonally across the field to the opposite corner, slowly jog along the end line to an adjacent corner, sprint diagonally across the field to the opposite corner, slowly jog along the end line back to your starting point. Repeat the circuit 3 to 5 times.

11. **Figure 8's.** Stand next to a goal on a regulation-size field. Sprint the length of the field, around the opposite goal, and return to the side of the goal opposite to where you started. The running pattern is a "figure 8." Rest for twice as long as it took you to run the "figure 8," then repeat the run. Complete 5 or more reps.

12. **Six-Step Ladder Run.** Begin on the midline of a regulation-size field. The steps of the ladder run are as follows:

    1. Jog to the 18 yard line.

    2. Sprint to the opposite 18 yard line.

    3. Jog to the midline.

    4. Sprint from the midline to the 6 yard line.

    5. Jog to the midline.

    6. Sprint to the end line.

    Rest for twice as long as it took you to complete the circuit, then repeat the run. Complete total of 4 to 6 repetitions.

# 5 Muscular Fitness

Strength training was once considered inappropriate for most athletes except for those in sports like competitive weight lifting, football, and wrestling. When I was playing professional soccer during the mid 1970's and early 1980's few players lifted weights. We just didn't see the benefit. We also had a misguided fear of becoming muscle bound and losing our flexibility. Since that time researchers have proved conclusively that my professional teammates and I were incorrect in our thinking. Sport scientists are in agreement that strength training should be an integral part of a soccer player's comprehensive fitness program. This applies to women, who have traditionally been excluded from weight training, as well as men. To play soccer successfully at a high level of competition requires muscular strength, explosive movement, sudden changes of speed and direction, and determined challenges for the ball. Each of these attributes can be improved through a soccer-specific weight training regimen, a program designed to develop total body strength, mus-

To play soccer successfully at a high level of competition requires muscular strength, explosive movement, sudden changes of speed and direction, and determined challenges for the ball. cular symmetry, balance, and coordination. Stronger muscles are also less likely to suffer injury, and if injury does occur, they recover more quickly than untrained muscles.

You must realize, however, that the ability to produce force during a soccer match is not entirely dependent on the strength of the muscles involved in the movement. Speed of movement is also a critical factor, as well as your ability to coordinate action of the movement . In other words, good timing is essential. It is important to recognize that just because you get stronger doesn't necessarily mean you will play better - but the odds are that you will.

## Components of Muscular Fitness

Muscular fitness can be divided into three primary components: muscular strength, muscular power, and muscular endurance. The combination of these distinct yet related components determine your overall level of muscular fitness.

### MUSCULAR STRENGTH

Strength is defined as the maximum force that a muscle or muscle group can exert in a single momentary contraction. For example, someone who can bench press 250 pounds has twice the strength of someone who can bench press 125 pounds. In this example strength is defined as the maximum weight the individual can lift one time. Your overall level of body strength, as well as the strength of individual muscles, is changeable and can be improved through training. Strength gains result from lifting heavy loads a few times (high weight - low reps) with the training effect being most noticeable in fast twitch muscle fibers.

Strength can be measured in several different ways. Dynamic strength is the most common method, and is defined as the maximal weight that can be lifted one time. Static strength is defined as the maximal amount of force that can be exerted against an immovable object. It is also referred to as isometric strength, and is specific to the angle at which the muscle(s) was trained. Static strength doesn't tell us much about strength throughout a range of motion, so it is not particularly applicable to sport performance. Isokinetic strength is a measure of force output throughout a range of motion. Soccer players, for the most part, will realize the greatest benefit from isokinetic strength training.

Strength training should be sport specific. For example, an Olympic power lifter will train in a different manner than would an endurance athlete. Your goal as a soccer player should be the development of functional strength - strength specific to the movements used in soccer. Functional strength training can be accomplished through the use of free weights, weight machines, manual resistance where a partner supplies the resistance, and also through soccer-related games where the typical movements used in a game are performed under conditions that are more stressful than normal.

> **Y**our overall level of body strength, as well as the strength of individual muscles, is changeable and can be improved through training.

### MUSCULAR ENDURANCE

Muscular endurance is a measure of a muscle's, or muscle group's, ability to sustain repeated movements. It is an essential fitness component in sports like soccer, basketball, and hockey that require repeated bouts of near-maximal or maximal efforts. Muscular endurance is developed by repetitive contractions of muscle fibers which in turn lead to changes in metabolic and circulatory patterns. There are different methods to improve muscular endurance. For example, to strengthen your quadricep (thigh) muscles you can do repeated leg extensions on a leg machine, or you can repeatedly shoot a soccer ball at maximum force off of a kick wall. Both types of exercise will improve muscular endurance, although the second method is more functional to the game of soccer.

The primary goals of muscle endurance training are to 1) improve the muscle's capacity to sustain intense activity, and 2) to decrease the recovery time needed by a muscle after intense exercise.

MUSCULAR POWER

By definition, power is the product of strength and speed of movement. It is the explosive aspect of strength, and provides a measure of how quickly you can display strength through a range of motion. Power is the rate of doing work.

$$power = (force \times distance) / time$$

In many sports, including soccer, power is actually more important than absolute strength. Your ability to perform explosive movements like jumping to outhead an opponent or accelerating into open space to receive the ball are, in part, dependent upon power. You can improve power by increasing strength, increasing speed of movement, or both. When training to develop power keep in mind the "principle of specificity" discussed earlier. Your training program should focus on the development of power specific to the game of soccer.

## The Training Stimulus

You should recall that improvements in fitness are related to the intensity, duration, and frequency of training. In Chapters 3 and 4 we discussed how the overload principle applies to aerobic and anaerobic fitness training. The same holds true when training to improve muscular fitness. The overload principle simply states that training workloads must impose a greater than normal demand, or overload, on our system in order to generate a training effect. As we become stronger additional workloads must be added in small increments to foster continued strength gains.

Strength training designed to improve absolute strength is best accomplished through a program of low repetitions with high weight. The physiological adaptations to such training include increased muscle size (hypertrophy) due to increases in contractile proteins and connective tissues, and possibly an increase in number of muscle fibers. In contrast, muscular endurance training is best accomplished through a program of high repetitions and low weight. Physiological adaptations to muscular endurance training include improved aerobic enzyme systems, increased number of mitochondria, and increased number of capillaries. These changes create more efficient aerobic pathways within the muscle fibers which in turn improve endurance.

## Prescriptions for Muscular Fitness Training

The strength training prescription is built around three variables: repetitions (reps), sets, and frequency. How these variables are manipulated will vary depending upon the specific objectives of the training.

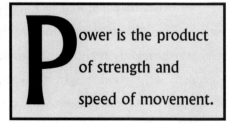

Power is the product of strength and speed of movement.

### REPETITIONS

To improve muscular strength you must involve as many muscle fibers as possible in a single movement. This can be accomplished by choosing a weight that you can lift 6 to 10 times in succession. Use lighter weights and perform more repetitions to improve muscular endurance.

### SETS

Three sets per exercise appears to be the optimal number for most athletes. Body builders and competitive weight lifters generally use more, and individuals who are just beginning a program can get results with less. One set may suffice if you are just beginning to strength train for the first time. Progress to two and then three sets as your strength improves.

### FREQUENCY

Three training sessions per week per muscle group appears to be the minimum frequency required to generate maximum gains in strength. Follow the hard-easy-hard format. A rest day should follow each workout. You must give your muscles sufficient time to recover from an intense strength workout. Cellular changes and improvements in strength actually occur during the rest days, not during the workouts.

## Strength Training for Kids?

A controversial issue among coaches, trainers, physicians, and parents involves the age at which young athletes should begin training with weights. In the past boys and girls were often discouraged from using free weights (dumbbells) due to fears that improper technique could result in damage to the growth center of developing bones. Concerns also centered around the potential for injury to connective tissues, and the belief that children lack sufficient levels of specific hormones needed to stimulate muscle development. Current research has done much to alleviate those fears, however, and has also demonstrated that children can improve strength through a properly supervised weight training program. The American College of Sports Medicine (ACSM) has joined with several other organizations to establish guidelines for weight training in preadolescent children. These guidelines include:

√ Adequate supervision by knowledgeable coaches.

√ All exercises should be performed through a full range of motion.

√ No maximum lifts should ever be attempted.

√ Training two or three sessions per week for 20 to 30 minutes per session is recommended.

√ Perform 6 to 15 repetitions per set. One to three sets per exercise is recommended.

√ Weight can be increased in one- to-three pound increments after the child can perform 15 repetitions in good form.

If free weights aren't readily available, boys and girls can use their own body weight as the resistance to be pushed or pulled. A variety of push-ups, pull-ups, dips, and abdominal exercises can provide the same strength benefits as weight training, and are equally beneficial for mature athletes as well.

## Sample Strength Training Program

There are no shortcuts to success. You cannot make significant strength gains overnight, or even during the two or three weeks prior to the season! Developing strength safely and effectively requires time, commitment, and hard work. The off-season is the best time of the year to make major improvements in your overall level of strength and muscular endurance. Once the playing season begins your fitness goals change from development of strength and endurance to maintenance.

To design a muscular fitness program that matches your needs and expectations, one that will reap the greatest performance benefits, you must take into account the following key elements:

√ Determine the specific muscular fitness requirements of competitive soccer.

√ Identify the major muscle groups involved.

√ Select exercises to develop total body muscular fitness.

√ Take into account individual strengths and weaknesses.

√ Establish a plan, set goals, and monitor your progress.

The following program is provided by Gary Wateska, head strength and conditioning coach for Olympic Sports at the University of Pittsburgh. Gary has worked with the Pittsburgh Steelers (NFL) and Pittsburgh Penguins (NHL), and is quite familiar with the muscular fitness needs of highly competitive athletes. The program is soccer-specific, covers a four-month training period, and focuses on the development of functional soccer strength. The primary goals of Gary's program are to 1) work every muscle in the body, 2) develop muscle symmetry, and 3) aid in injury prevention. For example, a common soccer injury is the strained hip flexor. A portion of this program is designed to strengthen hip flexors in order to prevent such injury.

Coach Wateska has provided two program options. The first is a total body workout performed three days per week with a rest day between workouts. Each workout takes about one hour of your time. The goal of the three-day option is to fatigue your whole body each time you work out. The program attempts to replicate as closely as possible the total body effort you must put forth in a game. In terms of time invested ( 3 hours per week), the three-day workout is very economical and efficient. Aerobic fitness training should occur on the rest days. The second option is a four days per week workout that focuses on different body parts on different days. On days #1 and #3 you will train legs, backs and biceps; on days #2 and #4 you train chest, shoulders, and triceps. The advantage of the four-day workout is that you can perform more exercises per body part in the same amount of time as the three-day program. However, you are also training one additional day per week. Regardless of which option you choose, abdominals should be trained every day.

You may choose to take advantage of both options. For example, you can use the three day per week program during months # 1 and #2, then switch to the four day per week program for months #3 and #4. In order to derive maximum benefit from these programs Coach Wateska stresses the following points:

√ Always warm up with light aerobic activity ( stationary bicycling, jogging, jumping rope) and stretching exercises prior to strength training.

√ Always work out with a partner or strength coach.

√ Weight training should not be a competition among teammates. Compete only with yourself, and progress at your own pace.

√ Work each muscle or muscle group through its full range of motion. This will help to improve flexibility as well as muscular strength.

√ Never sacrifice proper form for increased weight. Avoid bouncing the weight and arching your body.

√ Raise and lower the weight in a controlled manner.

√ Your goal is to reach momentary muscular fatigue at the end of each set. If you are not reaching muscular fatigue, the weight is probably too light.

√ Take a short rest between sets. The higher the intensity the more pronounced the results.

# Figure 5.1
## Three Day Per Week Workout

**DAY #1**

Neck Machine (1 set/10 reps - Front)
                  (1 set/10 reps - Back)
Squat/Leg Press (3 sets)
Leg Curl (3 sets)
Leg Extension (1 set/15 reps)
Hip Flexion (2 sets)
Bench Press (3 sets)
Dumbbell Incline (2 sets)
Front Pulldown (3 sets)
Cable Row (2 sets)
Shoulder Press (3 sets)
Lateral Raise (3 sets)
Straight Bar Curl (3 sets)
Tricep Pushdown (3 sets)

**DAY #2**

Pull-Ups (2 sets to fatigue)
Back Pulldown (3 sets)
Leverage Row (2 sets)
Pullover (2 sets)
Dumbbell Bench Press (3 sets)
Incline Bench (1 set/12 reps)
Dumbbell Flies (2 sets)
Dumbbell Shoulder Press (3 sets)
Upright Row (2 sets)
Rear Deltoids (2 sets)
Leg Extension (3 sets)
Leg Curl (3 sets)
Calf Raises (2 sets/15 reps)
Dips (2 sets to fatigue)

**DAY #3**

Neck Machine (1 set/10 reps - front)
 (1 set/10 reps - back)
Incline Bench Press (3 sets)
Bench Press (2 sets)
High Row (3 sets)
Dumbbell Row (3 sets)
Dumbbell Shoulder Press (2 sets)
Lateral Raise (2 sets)
Front Raise (2 sets)
Leg Press (3 sets)
Leg Curl (3 sets)
Hip Flexion (2 sets)
Bicep Curl (3 sets)
Tricep Pushdown (3 sets)
Push-Ups (1 set to fatigue)

**NOTE:** The above strength training program has been designed for mature, college-age athletes. Always consult with a knowledgeable strength and conditioning coach before beginning a program.

## Figure 5.2
## Four Day Per Week Workout

Days # 1 and #3 = Legs/Back/Biceps

ABDOMINALS EVERY DAY

Days # 2 and #4 = Chest/Shoulders/Triceps

Neck Exercises = 2 days (Your choice)

### DAY #1

Leg Press/Squat (3 sets)

Leg Curl (3 sets)

Leg Extension (1 set/15 reps)

Adduction (2 sets)

Calf Raises ( 3 sets)

Hip Flexion (2 sets)

Front Pulldown (3 sets)

Cable Row (3 sets)

Pullover (2 sets)

Low Back Exercise (2 sets/12 reps)

Straight Bar Curl (2 sets)

Dumbbell Curl (2 sets)

Preacher Curl (2 sets)

### DAY #2

Bench Press (3 sets)

Dumbbell Incline Press (3 sets)

Dumbbell Flies (2 sets)

Shoulder Press (3 sets)

Upright Row (1 set/15 reps)

Lateral Raise (2 sets)

Rear Deltoids (2 sets)

Tricep Pushdown (3 sets)

Push-Ups (2 sets to fatigue)

Dips (2 sets to fatigue)

### DAY #3

Pull-Ups (2 sets to fatigue)

Back Pulldown (3 sets)

High Row (3 sets)

Front Pulldown (1 set /15 reps)

Dumbbell Row (2 sets)

Low Back (1 set/12 reps)

Leg Press (3 sets)

Leg Extension (2 sets)

Leg Curl (3 sets)

Hip Flexion (1 set)

Calf Raise (1 set/25 reps)

Straight Bar Curl (3 sets)

Dumbbell Incline Curl (2 sets)

### DAY #4

Dumbbell Bench Press (3 sets)

Bench Press (1 set/15 reps)

Incline Bench (2 sets)

Peck Deck (2 sets)

Dumbbell Shoulder Press (3 sets)

Lateral Raise (2 sets)

Front Raise (2 sets)

Rear Deltoid (2 sets)

French Curl (3 sets)

Dumbbell Tricep Extension (2 sets)

Bench Dips (2 sets to fatigue)

**NOTE:** The above strength training program has been designed for mature, college-age athletes. Always consult with a knowledgeable strength and conditioning coach before beginning a program.

NOTE: Unless otherwise noted, the number of repetitions per set for both the three- and four-day workout programs is as follows:

(Warm-up sets are not included in the required number of sets)

Month #1: 3-set exercises: 12 reps/10 reps/10 reps

2-set exercises: 10 reps/10 reps

Month #2: 3-set exercises: 10 reps/10 reps/8 reps

2-set exercises: 10 reps/8 reps

Month #3: 3-set exercises: 10 reps/8 reps/6 reps

2-set exercises: 8 reps/8 reps

Month #4: 3-set exercises: 10 reps/6 reps/ 6 reps

2-set exercises: 8 reps/6 reps

# 6 Strength Training Exercises

A variety of exercises can be used to improve strength. Some utilize fitness machines such as Nautilus, Universal and Hammer Strength. Others rely on free weights and dumbbells as the resistance to be moved. If equipment isn't available, manual resistance supplied by a training partner or even the resistance of your own body weight can produce virtually the same results. The key to improving strength doesn't hinge on fancy machines or the type of resistance that you move, but rather on the effort and commitment you put into your workouts. As we've said before, there are no shortcuts to success.

The following pages describe and illustrate many of the strength training exercises listed in the program provided by coach Gary Wateska in Chapter 5. Exercises are grouped according to the major muscles involved.

**REMEMBER:** A spotter (training partner) should be used for all free weight exercises.

## Chest

### STRAIGHT BAR BENCH PRESS

Lie on bench so that your shoulders and buttocks are in contact with the bench. Plant feet firmly on ground. Place your hands on the bar about 6 inches wider than shoulder width in an overhand grip. Lift off with spotter and gain control of the bar. Slowly lower the bar to your chest. Push weight up until elbows are locked. Do not bounce weight off of chest, and never raise buttocks off of bench. Inhale while lowering, exhale while raising.

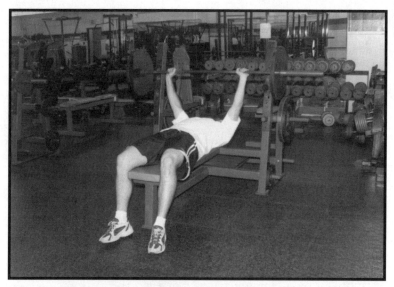

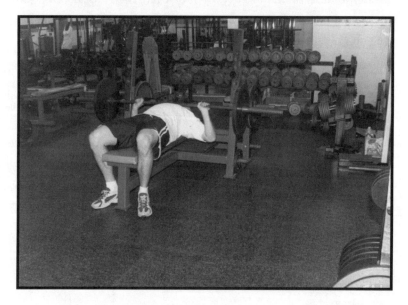

**DUMBBELL BENCH PRESS**

Lie on bench with feet flat on floor. Hold dumbbells at arms length directly above shoulders with palms facing forward. Slowly lower the dumbbells until they are even with and 12 inches to each side of your chest . Return dumbbells to starting position using same path. Inhale while lowering, exhale while raising.

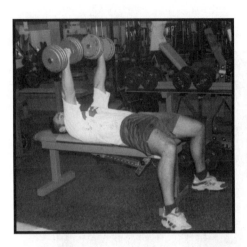 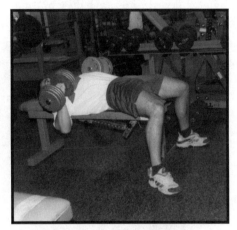

**STRAIGHT BAR INCLINE BENCH PRESS**

Grasp bar with hands slightly wider than shoulder width apart. Keep your back flat against incline bench with feet firmly planted. Lift off with spotter and position weight directly above upper chest. Slowly lower weight to chest just above the nipple line. Pause, focus eyes upward, drive through legs, and push weight up to start position. Keep head on bench, do not arch back too sharply. Do not raise hips off of bench.

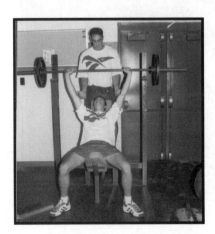 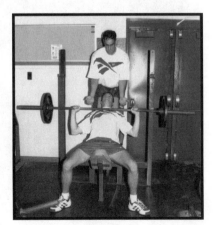

DUMBBELL INCLINE BENCH PRESS

Lie on 45-degree incline bench with head and hips on bench and feet firmly planted on ground. Begin with dumbbells positioned even with shoulders in full stretched position with palms facing forward. Raise the weight straight up above upper chest, pause, and then lower weight to chest in a slow, controlled movement. Arms should be close at all times. Do not bounce weight off of chest when lowering. Inhale while lowering, exhale while raising.

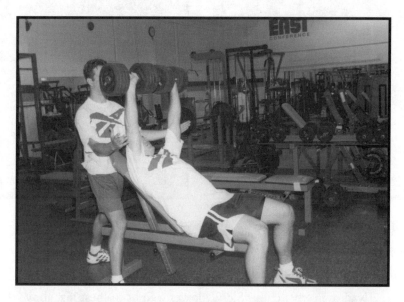

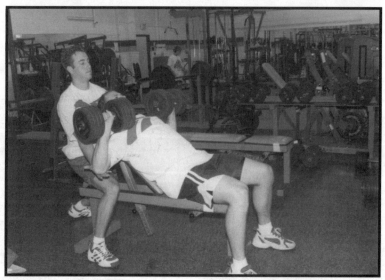

**PUSH-UPS**

Assume a push-up position with arms approximately shoulder-width apart and legs straight behind. Slowly lower your body until your chest contacts the ground, then use your arms to rise to the starting position. Keep your back straight and head up. Do not let your body sag. Inhale while lowering, exhale while raising. Repeat as many times as possible.

For variation do 1) push-ups with hands placed on top of soccer ball, 2) push-ups with feet positioned on flat bench.

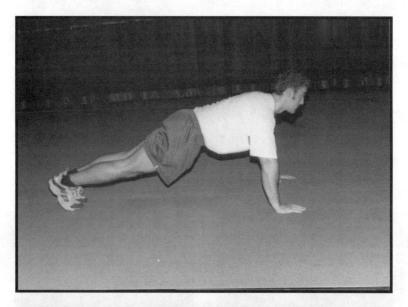

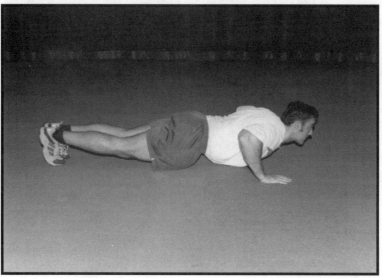

## DIPS

Support yourself by grabbing bars with an overhand grip and palms facing each other. Keep your arms straight. Lower your body by bending shoulders and elbows until elbows are bent at 90 degrees, pause, and return to starting position. Inhale while lowering, exhale while raising. Do not swing body back and forth. Perform as many reps as possible.

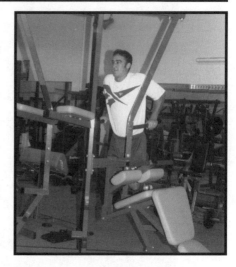

## BENCH DIPS

Support body weight on edge of bench with arms extended, palms facing down, and fingers pointing behind you. Keep legs straight with heels on level surface. Slowly lower body by bending at the elbows, pause, and then raise to the starting position. Perform as many reps as possible.

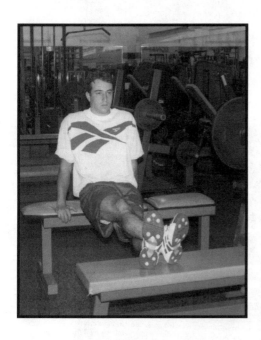
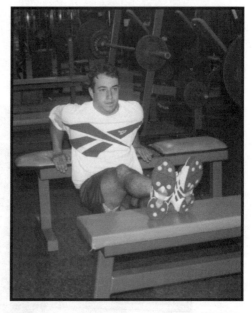

# SHOULDERS

### STRAIGHT BAR SHOULDER PRESS

Sit on military bench with back straight. Grasp bar with an overhand grip slightly wider than shoulder width. Begin with bar on upper chest. Drive through the legs and lift bar straight up. Press bar to arms length overhead. Pause for a moment, then slowly return bar to upper chest position. Rest the bar on your chest between reps. Note: The shoulder press can also be done from a standing position.

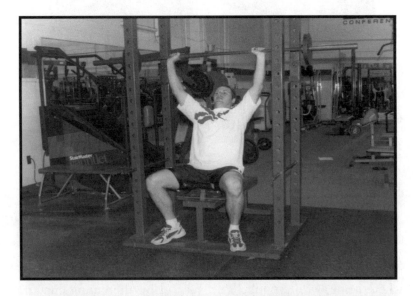

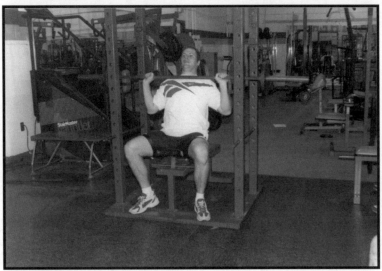

### SEATED DUMBBELL SHOULDER PRESS

Sit on bench with feet firmly on floor. Raise dumbbells to shoulder height. Keep elbows out, thumbs facing in, palms facing forward. Press dumbbells upward to arms length overhead, pause, and lower weights to starting position. Can also be done when standing, with palms facing in or out.

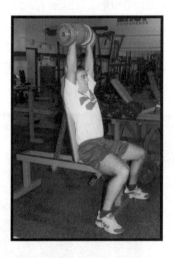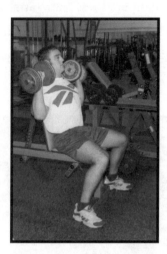

### DUMBBELL FRONT RAISE

Stand holding dumbbells in front of thighs with palms facing in. Position feet shoulder width apart with body erect and knees slightly bent. Keep your arms and elbows slightly bent, and raise dumbbells in an arc until your arms are parallel to floor. Return dumbbells to starting position using same path. This exercise can also be done when sitting, with dumbbells at sides, or by alternating one arm up, one arm down.

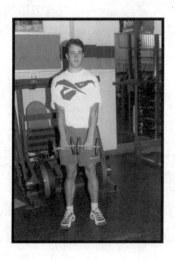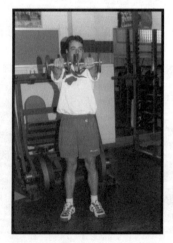

### LATERAL RAISE

Stand erect with arms extended straight down to sides. Hold dumbbells with palms facing in. Raise dumbbells in a semicircular motion to slightly above shoulder height, pause, and then lower dumbbells to starting position using the same pathway. Keep arms straight as you raise the dumbbells. Inhale while lowering, exhale while raising.

**Variation on machine:** Sit in machine, fasten belt, place arms in handles. Make sure elbows are slightly behind torso and against pads. Raise elbows slowly to chin level, pause, and return to starting position.

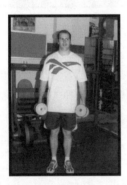 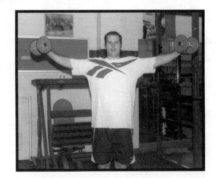

### DUMBBELL REAR DELT RAISE

Bend forward at the waist with your forehead at approximately waist height. Hold dumbbells with arms extended down and elbows locked. Slowly raise dumbbells to shoulder height, even with ears, and momentarily hold that position. Do not swing dumbbells upward. Slowly lower dumbbells to starting position.

**Variation on Nautilus machine:** Sit with arms crossed and triceps contacting pads. Bend arms in a rowing movement as far back as possible, pause, and return slowly to the starting position. Keep arms parallel to the floor.

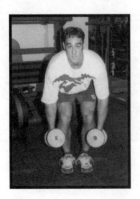 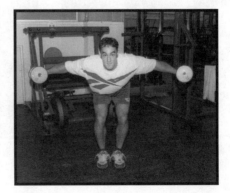

## Back

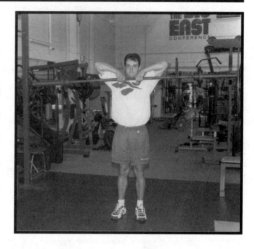

### UPRIGHT ROW

Hold bar with hands in an overhand grip several inches apart. With knees slightly bent and body erect, pull weight up to chin position. Elbows should be even with or higher than the bar. Slowly return weight to starting point, pause and repeat.

### MEDIUM GRIP PULL-UPS

Grab overhead bar with overhand grip and hands approximately shoulder width apart. Relax legs and keep them straight beneath you. Pull your body upward until chin is even with the bar, then slowly lower yourself to the starting position. Do not swing back and forth. Repeat as many times as possible.

**Note:** Variations include close grip, wide grip, reverse grip (palms facing inward) pull-ups.

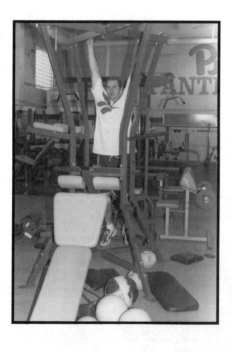 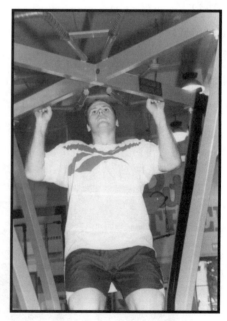

**REAR LAT PULL-DOWN**

Sit on bench facing machine. Grasp bar with an overhand grip and hands wider than shoulder width apart. Pull bar straight down until it touches the base of your neck just above the shoulders. Pause, slowly return to starting position, and repeat. Inhale while lowering, exhale while raising. This exercise can also be done with medium width grip.

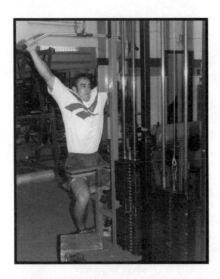 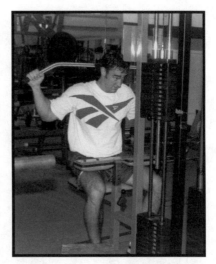

**FRONT PULL-DOWN**

Sit on bench facing machine. Hold bar in an overhand grip with hands approximately shoulder width apart. Pull bar down in front of face until even with upper chest. Pause, return to starting position. Inhale while lowering, exhale while raising.

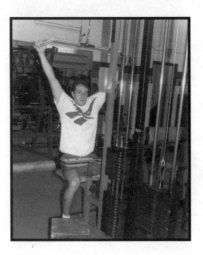 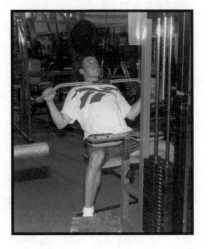

CABLE ROW

Sit facing machine with knees flexed and feet against the support platform. Lean forward and grab the cable handle with arms fully extended. Pull the cable handle to the sides of your chest in line with pectorals. Pause, then slowly extend arms to starting position. This exercise can also be done one arm at a time.

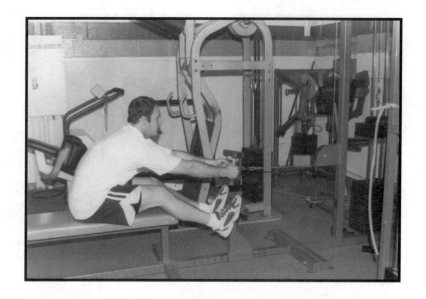

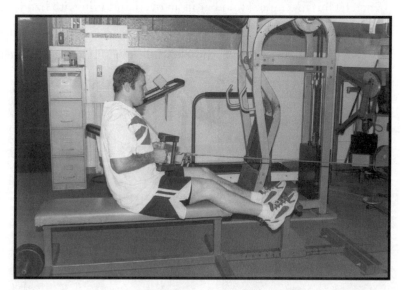

## HIGH ROW

Sit on machine with back toward weights. Adjust the seat so that your arms must be fully extended to reach handles. Keep your back straight and your chest against the pad at all times. Slowly pull handles to chest, pause, then slowly extend arms to full stretch position.

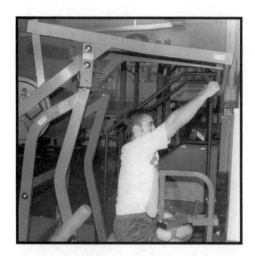 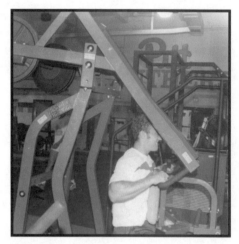

## LEVERAGE ROW

Sit on leverage row machine facing the hand grips. Adjust seat so your arms are parallel to the floor when reaching for the handles. Keep chest against pad at all times. Pull handles to chest, pause, then slowly extend arms to full stretch position.

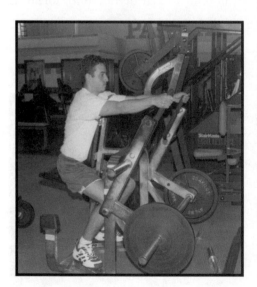 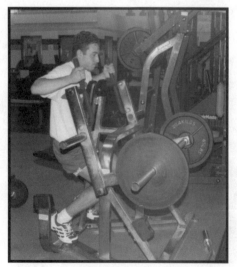

## PULLOVER

Sit in machine and fasten seat belt. Place elbows on pads behind your head with hands against the movement arm. Exert pulldown force with elbows, not hands. Pull the movement arm to your midsection during every repetition, then slowly return to starting position (elbows near or slightly past your head).

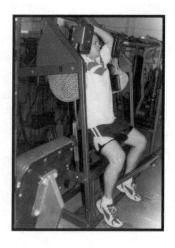 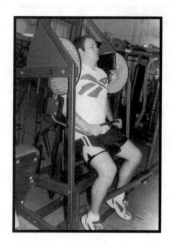

## Arms

### STRAIGHT BAR CURL

Hold bar with hands approximately 12 inches apart and palms facing up. Stand erect, back straight, head up and feet shoulder width apart. Begin with bar at arms length resting against upper thighs. Curl bar in semicircular motion until forearms touch biceps. Keep elbows in and upper arms close to sides. Lower bar using same path. Inhale while lowering, exhale while raising. Do not swing arms or arch back to help lift weight.

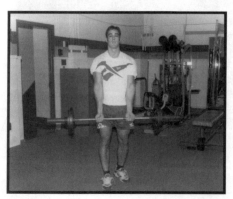 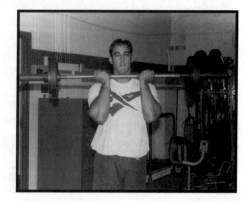

PREACHER CURL

Sit facing forward on preacher bench with chest and arms against the pad. Extend upper pectorals over the end of bench, and hold bar with both hands approximately 15 inches apart. Keep upper arms against pad. Start with bar at arms length, curl bar in semicircular motion until forearms touch biceps. Return to starting position using same path. Do not let the elbows go beyond full extension position. Inhale while lowering, exhale while raising.

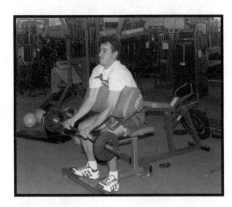 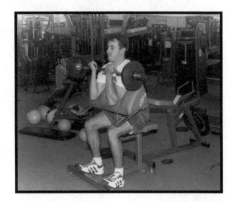

FRENCH CURL

Lie flat on your back on a bench. Grasp the curl bar with palms facing up and hands approximately thumbs distance apart. Extend arms to full length directly above chest. Keep upper arms perpendicular to the bench as you bend at the elbows and lower bar to a position just above your forehead. Pause, then slowly return bar to the starting position. All movement should originate from flexion at the elbows.

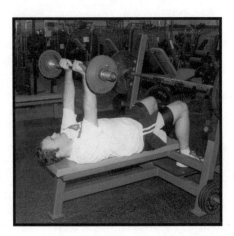 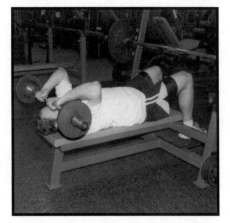

### TRICEP PUSH-DOWN

Stand erect facing bar. Take a close overhand grip with elbows in tight and bar at mid-chest height. Extend arms and press bar down until elbows lock. Slowly return weight to starting position, pause, and repeat. Elbows should remain motionless throughout the movement. Avoid leaning forward into the bar.

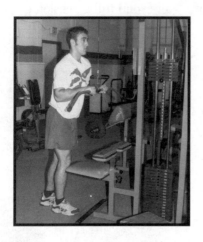 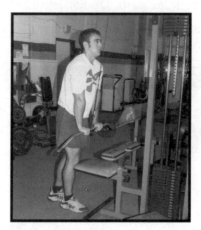

## LEGS/HIPS

### LEG PRESS

Place feet about shoulder width apart in a comfortable position on the foot plate. Keep your back flat against the pad and hold the hand grips. Bring weight down until thighs near chest. The angle between your upper and lower leg should be about 90 degrees. Push weight up just short of locking knees, pause, and then re-peat. Inhale while lowering, exhale while raising. Do not bounce at bottom position, do not bring knees together on the way up.

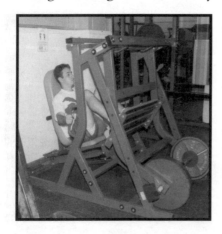 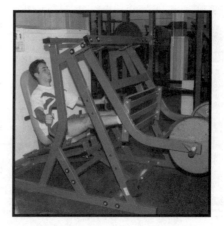

## LEG EXTENSION

Sit on a leg machine with your knee joint slightly over the edge of the bench. Place feet under lower foot pads. Grasp seat or handles if provided. Keep buttocks down and simultaneously extend both legs to full extension. Pause, return to full bent position, and repeat.

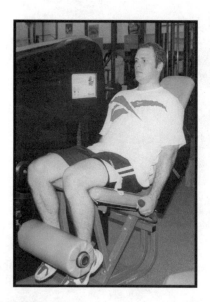 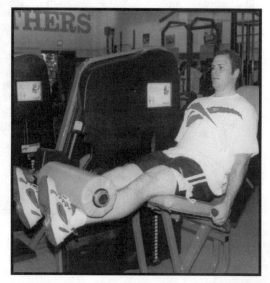

## LEG CURL

Lie face down with knee caps slightly over the edge of the bench. Place heels under pads, hold side handles or side of bench. Keep hips down, and slowly curl the weight to your buttocks. Pause for a moment, then slowly lower the weight to full leg extension. Can be done one leg at a time or both legs at a time.

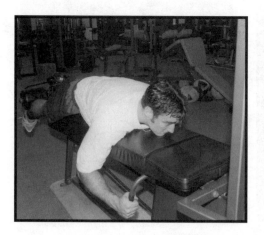 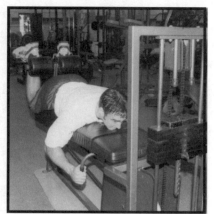

SEATED CALF RAISE

Sit with feet together on the machine. Begin in a full stretched position with heels positioned diagonally downward toward floor. Extend forward on toes as far as possible, pause, and slowly return to the full stretched position.

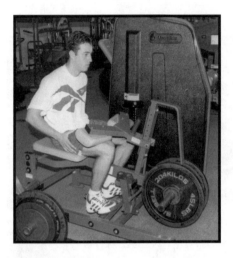 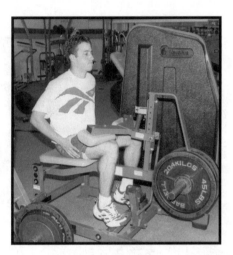

HIP FLEXION

Adjust floorboard on machine so that hip joint is lined up with axis of the cam. The knee pad should contact your leg just above the knee. Simulate a running motion while keeping constant tension on the muscle being worked. Work one leg at a time.

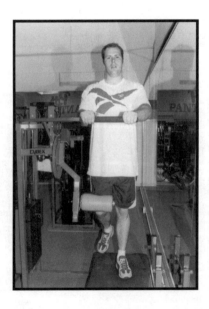 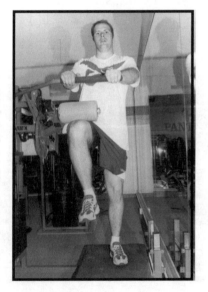

# Neck

### SEATED NECK EXTENSION AND FLEXION

Select desired weight on neck machine. Sit with upper body erect. Position forehead against pad. Look up with neck in stretched position. Extend head forward until you are looking at the floor. Pause, then slowly return to starting position. Do not lean forward or back when lowering and raising head. Repeat with back of head against pad.

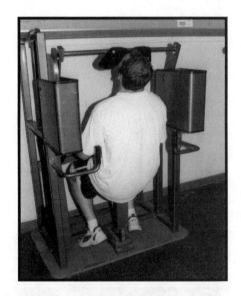

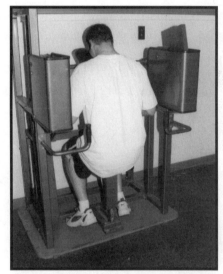

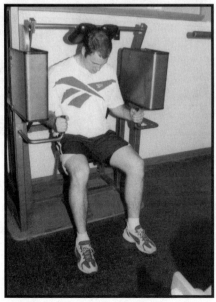

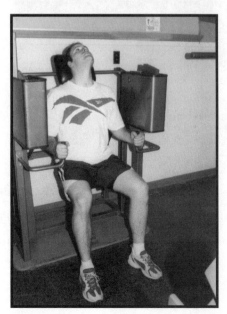

SEATED PARTNER-SYSTEM NECK RESISTANCE

Sit on end of bench. Cross arms, keep back straight and head up. Partner puts a towel over your head to keep head from slipping.

> **Exercise #1.** Partner stands behind you while straddling a bench with hands on your forehead. Pull your head forward as partner applies resistance.

> **Exercise #2.** Partner places hands behind your head. Push your head back as partner supplies resistance to movement.

> **Exercise #3.** Partner places hands to right side of your head. Push your head to the right as partner supplies resistance.

> **Exercise #4.** Partner places hands to left side of your head. Push your head to the left as partner supplies resistance.

## Abdominal Exercises

CRUNCHES

Lie flat on your back with knees flexed and arms folded across chest. Rise slowly until upper back is at a 45-degree angle with floor. Lower yourself slowly to ground and repeat. Perform 20 to 30 reps.

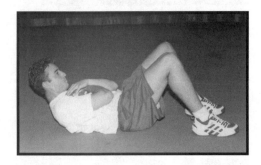 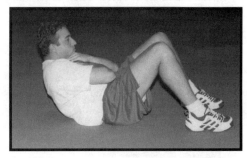

WALL SIT-UPS

Sit with your legs extended diagonally upward against the waist of a standing partner (or a wall) . Keep your legs straight as you sit up and touch your hands to your toes. Repeat as many times as possible.

### INCLINE LEG PULL-IN

Position sit-up board upward at a 30- to 35-degree angle. Lie on the board with your head at the top; hold the bar behind your head with both hands. Bend knees, pulling your upper thighs into your midsection. Return to starting position and then repeat. Do not let your heels touch the board once you have begun the exercise. To make the exercise more difficult, hold a light dumbbell between your feet.

### FLAT BENCH WEIGHTED LEG RAISE

Lie on a flat bench with legs extended over the end. Place hands under buttocks with palms down. Keep knees locked and legs straight. Raise legs as high as possible. Lower legs until they are about 6 inches off of the floor. To increase difficulty position a light weight between your feet.

# 7 Speed Training

As the level of competition increases, so does the speed of play. When coaches talk of speed of play they are speaking about much more than your ability to run fast, however. Granted, absolute (sprinting) speed is one element of the mix, but of equal importance are a number of other factors. Quickness of movement, speed with the ball, speed of skill execution, directional speed, and speed of decision-making all impact soccer performance, as does the ability to accelerate quickly from different positions. With respect to the game of soccer, speed is a complex concept.

## Speed Without the Ball

### ABSOLUTE SPEED

Your ability to run fast is, for the most part, genetically determined. To be a great sprinter you must pick your parents well! If you have been blessed with a preponderance of fast twitch (explosive) muscle fiber , then there is a good chance that you are a fast runner, or at least possess the physical potential to be a fast runner. On the other hand, if you were born with a high percentage of slow twitch (endurance) muscle fiber, your chances of becoming an Olympic sprinter are very slim. That being said, don't be discouraged if you aren't a fast runner by nature's design. The fact remains that absolute sprinting speed, although important, is not the most important aspect of soccer-specific speed. Rarely during a game is a player required to go straight ahead for any significant distance without having to change speed, direction or both.

You can improve absolute speed to a limited extent through speed training. Gains in speed are generally due to improved leg strength and power, as well as to improved running mechanics. Methods used to improve absolute speed can be lumped into two general categories: 1) sprint resistance training, and 2) sprint assisted training. The first category involves sprint running performed against a resistance. The goal of sprint resistance training is the improvement of dynamic strength. Popular training methods include uphill running and parachute running. Sprint assisted training is designed to improve leg speed movement. Methods of training include downhill running, sprinting on a motor-driven treadmill at speeds greater than those during actual sprint running, and towing behind an automobile at speeds above maximum unassisted speed. (Note: Do not use auto towing method unless supervised by a knowledgeable trainer or coach).

You can also improve your running speed by improving your flexibility. This is especially true if you are tightly muscled and inflexible to begin with. By improving dynamic flexibility you can lengthen your stride which enables your muscles to work through a more complete range of motion. This, in turn, allows for increased leg speed as well as increases in the potential force developed.

The majority of speed training can occur during regular practice sessions. Keep in mind, however, that it is difficult to improve speed when you are in a fatigued state that diminishes correct form and running technique. For that reason, speed training should be performed when you are relatively fresh, preferably early in the training session. It is also important to allow your energy systems time to recover fully between sprints. This will ensure that you are performing "quality" rather than "quantity" training. The recovery time needed will vary from one athlete to the next depending upon level of fitness and intensity of the work interval.

Vern Gambetta, a nationally recognized conditioning expert and speed training specialist, believes that three elements constitute good sprint mechanics: Posture, Arm Action, and Leg Action. When running at top speed you should carry your body in a relatively erect posture. Your arm action should be smooth and rhythmic. Proper arm action will help in controlling your stride. The leg action differs from that used for acceleration runs in the sense that, instead of pushing off of the ground with each step, you are essentially running over the ground. A careful blend of stride length and stride frequency is the key to achieving maximum sprinting speed. The relatively long stride length used when sprinting over longer distances is not par-

ticularly suited to successful soccer performance. A more compact stride that emphasizes leg speed provides greater control and enhances your ability to suddenly change speed and direction. Full extension of the knee should not occur when sprinting. Consider the following points when training to improve absolute sprinting speed:

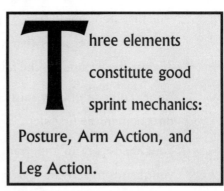

Three elements constitute good sprint mechanics: Posture, Arm Action, and Leg Action.

√ Allow sufficient recovery between repetitions.

√ Sprint training should be done early in the practice session, preferably after the warm-up.

√ Interval training can be used to improve running technique as well as fitness.

√ Include a ball in running drills whenever possible so increases in speed can transfer to the game.

√ Pay close attention to detail. Economy of movement and effective use of the arms are essential. Not only is arm movement important for straight-ahead speed, it also initiates changes in direction.

DIRECTIONAL SPEED

Soccer is a game of quick starts and sudden stops interspersed with constant changes of speed and direction. These types of movements, often referred to as directional speed or speed off-the-mark, can be enhanced through strength training, plyometric (jump training), and also by improved running mechanics. According to Vern Gambetta, several simple mechanical principles must be followed in order to improve quickness off-the-mark:

1. Your first step is critical – it must be in the desired direction of movement. A common mistake is a miss-step, or false step, away from the intended direction of movement.

2. The first step should be lower to the ground than each succeeding step. This ensures that you are in proper position to push against the ground on the following steps.

3. Your center of gravity must move horizontally in the intended direction on the first step. It should not move up or down.

4. Your hands play an important role in initiating movement. Move your hands to activate a vigorous arm thrust.

Practice directional speed from a variety of starting positions. For example, begin with feet in a staggered position with one positioned forward of the other, or facing opposite the intended direction of movement (as with a checking run), or when jumping as if trying to out-jump an opponent to head the ball. Once you have become comfortable with the running mechanics, include a ball in your training.

ACCELERATION SPEED

Acceleration speed refers to your ability to reach maximum speed in the shortest time possible. Soccer players must be able to rapidly accelerate to full speed over distances as short as 10 to 15 yards. You can improve acceleration speed through the following exercises.

*Follow the Leader Run*

Pair with a teammate. He or she runs in random fashion throughout a large field area while constantly changing speed and direction. You follow closely and try to shadow, or imitate, his or her running patterns while maintaining a distance of two yards or less.

### Resistance Runs

Run at top speed against resistance. The resistance can be provided by running up hills, and also by pulling a parachute.

### Acceleration Sprints

Over a distance of 45 yards, jog the first 15 yards, run the middle segment at three-quarter speed, and sprint the last 15 yards. After crossing the finish line gradually slow to a jog, return to the starting line, and repeat.

## Speed With the Ball

Speed without the ball is just one aspect of soccer-specific speed. Speed with the ball, often referred to as technical speed, is actually more critical to overall performance. The ability to quickly pass, receive, shoot and dribble under the pressures of game competition can save precious moments and actually make you a "faster" player. Your first touch of the ball is always the most important touch you will get, because that is the time when you either gain or lose precious seconds. Your first touch must always prepare the ball for your second touch , or your next intended movement.

Great technical speed in and of itself does not guarantee superior performance however. For example, even though you may possess exceptional passing skills your overall performance will suffer if you consistently make poor decisions in the heat of competition (i.e., hold the ball too long before passing, dribble into defensive pressure, choose the poorest passing option). To succeed at the highest levels of competition you must couple a high level of technical speed with the ability to make effective, split-second decisions in response to constantly changing game situations. This ability is commonly referred to as your tactical speed. You can improve both technical and tactical speed through a variety of skill-related drills and small-group exercises. The following progression of drills is provided to illustrate how you can improve your speed with the ball as well as your decision-making speed. The drills can be modified to suit the age and ability of players.

DRILL #1. NUMBERS PASSING GAME (AS WARM-UP)

Organize into groups of four. Number each player in the group beginning with #1 and continuing through #4. Play in an area of 15 by 25 yards. Players #1 and #3 each have possession of a ball to begin. All players jog randomly within the area; those with a ball dribble it. The dribblers locate the teammate numbered directly above and pass to him or her. Player #4 always passes to player #1 to complete the circuit. All players move continuously for the duration of the drill as they pass to the teammate numbered above and receive passes from the teammate numbered below.

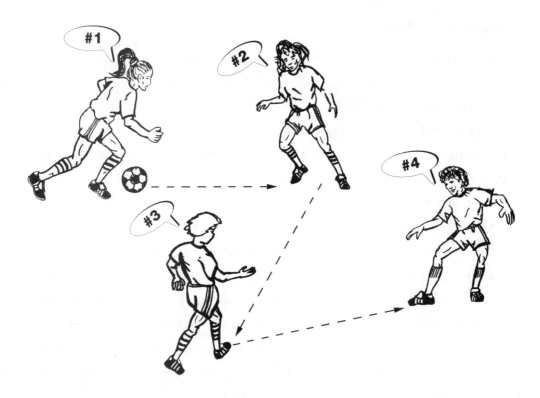

### DRILL #2 THREE VERSUS ONE IN GRID

Use cones to mark a 12 yards square. Divide into groups of four. Designate 3 players as attackers and 1 as the defender in each group. The attackers attempt to keep the ball from the defender by passing among themselves within the square. If the defender steals the ball, or kicks it out of the square, he or she immediately returns it to one of the attackers and play continues. Play for 4 minutes, then designate a different player as the defender. Award the attacking team 1 point for eight consecutive passes without possession loss. Award the defender 1 point for each time he or she steals the ball, or causes the attackers to play the ball out of the grid. The presence of a defender in this drill forces the attackers to make more decisions (i.e., where and when to pass the ball) and shifts the focus from purely technical speed to also include tactical decision-making speed.

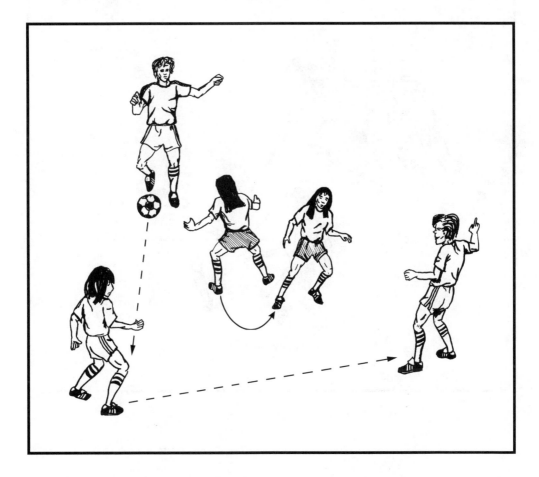

DRILL #3 THREE VERSUS TWO IN GRID

Increase the field size to 12 by 15 yards. Three attackers attempt to keep the ball from two defenders within the area. Award points in the same manner as in Drill #2. The addition of a second defender reduces the available space and requires the attackers to increase their speed of play from both a technical and tactical standpoint. It also magnifies the relative importance of each decision because there is less margin for error. Play for 10 minutes, then designate two different defenders.

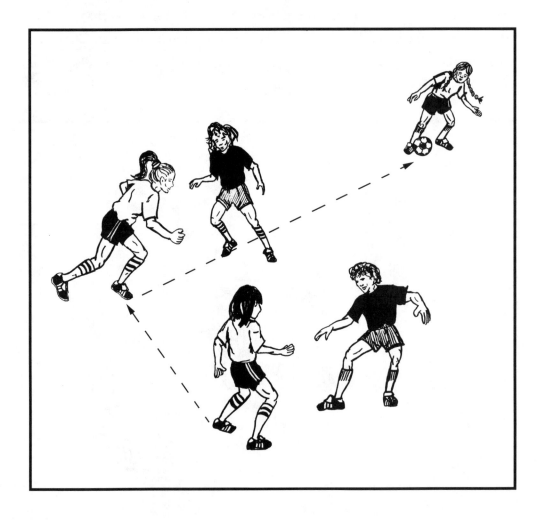

### DRILL #4 THREE VERSUS THREE (PLUS 1 NEUTRAL)

Increase the playing area size to 20 by 25 yards. Designate two teams of 3 players each plus 1 neutral player who always joins the team with possession to create a 4 versus 3 player advantage. Use colored scrimmage vests to differentiate teams and the neutral player. Award one team possession of the ball to begin. Change of possession occurs when a defending player steals the ball, or when the ball goes out of play last touched by a member of the attacking team. Award 1 team point for 6 consecutive passes without possession loss. Play for 15 minutes. The team scoring the most points wins.

By adding players to the drill we have reduced the available space and time which forces the players to increase speed of play as well as speed of decision-making. Virtually all of the pressures encountered in actual match competition (player movement, compacted space, limited time, physical fatigue, challenging opponents) are represented in this drill.

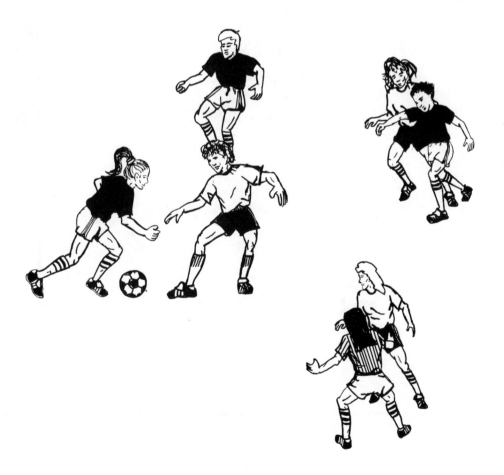

### DRILL #5 THREE VERSUS THREE GAME (MICRO-SOCCER)

Use cones to mark off a field 25 by 30 yards. Position a goal at the center of each end line. Designate two teams of three players each. Each team defends a goal and can score in the opponent's goal. Do not use goalkeepers. Points are scored in two ways: 1) eight consecutive passes without loss of possession scores 1 team point, and/or 2) shooting the ball into the opponent's goal scores 2 team points.

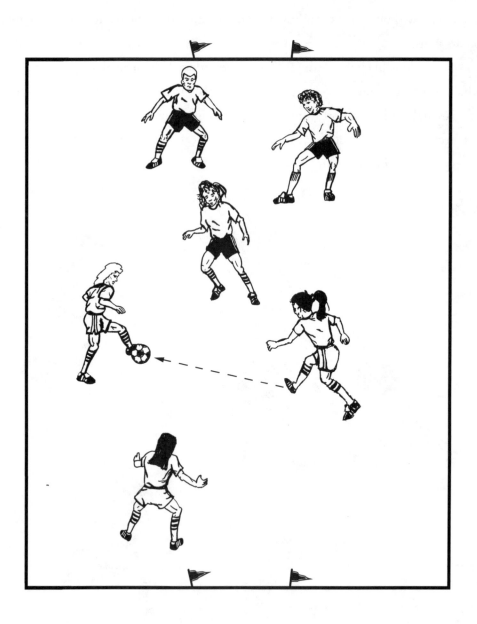

Small-sided games provide an ideal training environment for developing speed with the ball. Players touch the ball more often than they would in a full-sided (11 versus 11) game, they are required to make decisions more frequently, and they must do so under the game-simulated pressures of restricted time and space. Obviously, as with any form of fitness training, each player must challenge himself or herself to the fullest extent to realize maximum benefits.

# 8 Flexibility and Agility Training

Flexibility and agility are related components of muscular fitness. Both attributes deal with movement ability, flexibility more so with individual body parts, whereas agility deals with movement of the body as a whole. You can improve both flexibility and agility through proper training.

## Flexibility

Flexibility can be defined as the range of possible movement around a joint or series of joints. It is an important aspect of athletic performance, particularly in sports like soccer that require finely skilled movements. Poor flexibility will inhibit your ability to perform skills, and also increases the likelihood of muscular and connective tissue injury. The range of movement around a particular joint can be limited by factors that are out of your control. For example, the boney structure of your elbows and knees sets definite limits on flexibility in those areas. Movement around other joints, such as the ankle and hip, is restricted by softer tissues like tendons and ligaments, muscles, joint capsules, and even the skin. In joints where movement is limited by soft tissues we can improve our range of motion through stretching exercises.

### IMPROVING FLEXIBILITY

The old adage "use it or lose it" definitely applies to flexibility. If you don't make a conscious effort to maintain flexibility, particularly as you get older, your range of motion will gradually decrease. Historically, two types of stretching exercises have been popular with coaches and trainers. The conventional method of stretching involves bouncing or bobbing motions that gradually extend the muscle(s) to greater and greater lengths. This method is commonly referred to as ballistic stretching. A common ballistic stretch is straight leg toe-touches where you gradually try to extend your hands closer to the floor through a rhythmic up-and-down bouncing motion. The alternative method of improving flexibility is called static stretching. Rather than using bouncing movements to elongate the muscle, static stretches slowly extend the target muscle or group of muscles to its greatest possible length without discomfort.

> If you don't make a conscious effort to maintain flexibility, particularly as you get older, your range of motion will gradually decrease.

Hold the stretch for 15 to 30 seconds, relax, and then move into a deeper stretch for an additional 15 to 30 seconds. Repeat each stretch a minimum of two times. Although both types of stretching can improve your flexibility, sport scientists are in agreement that static stretching is the preferred method. Static stretching is equally if not more effective than ballistic stretching for increasing range of motion, and as an added benefit it is much safer because your muscles aren't subjected to the sudden pressures and strains imposed by bouncing movements. A slow and steady extension of the muscle also inhibits firing of the stretch reflex, the body's built-in safeguard against overextending. In contrast, the bouncing movements of ballistic stretching usually activate the stretch reflex which opposes your efforts to stretch the muscle.

For optimal results stretch every day, or at the very least, every other day. The best times to stretch are before and after each workout. Never stretch a cold muscle. Five to ten minutes of light work with the ball prior to stretching will elevate muscle temperatures and promote increased blood flow. This in turn improves muscle suppleness and helps to prevent next day soreness. Don't expect to see major improvements in flexibility overnight. It generally takes three to five weeks of regular stretching to realize significant changes.

Individuals may vary greatly in the extent of their flexibility, so you should always measure progress against your own standards and initial state of flexibility. Stretching should never become an arena for competition among teammates. Your goal is to improve flexibility in a safe, injury-free manner, not to outstretch your buddies. It is safe to say, however, that although not everyone has the same flexibility, everyone can improve their flexibility.

## Flexibility (Static Stretch) Exercises

The major muscle groups used in soccer include the hamstrings, quadriceps, calves, groin, lower back, upper torso, neck, and shoulders. Use the following exercises to improve your flexibility. Be sure to hold the stretch position for 15 to 30 seconds, and repeat each stretch at least twice.

**HAMSTRINGS**

### Straight Leg Sit

Sit on the floor with legs extended in front of you. Keep legs straight and together. Lean forward with arms extended and try to touch your toes.

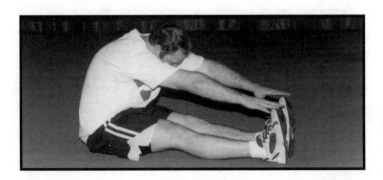

*Sitting Hamstring Stretch*

Assume a sitting position with your left leg straight and right leg bent 90 degrees. Position the heel of the right foot against the inside of the left thigh. Keep your left leg straight as you bend forward at the waist and attempt to touch your left foot. Repeat with opposite leg.

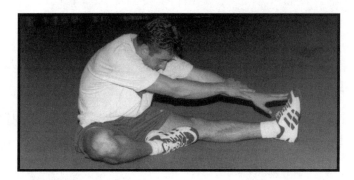

*Bent Leg Hamstring Stretch*

Sit with knees bent and feet flat on the ground. Place your right hand behind your left ankle and your left hand behind your left thigh. Flex at the hip and pull gently on your calf until you feel tension. Repeat using your right leg.

*Split Leg Stretch*

Assume a sitting position with legs spread at an angle of approximately 45 degrees. Lower your head toward your right knee, then repeat to the left knee. Try to keep your back straight and your stomach muscles tight.

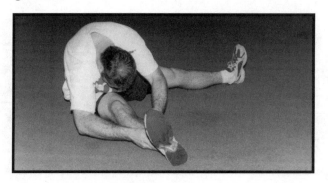

QUADRICEPS

*Lying on Side Quad Stretch*

Lie on your left side, using your left forearm for support. Flex your right leg and grab your right ankle with your right hand. Slowly pull your leg back until you feel tension in your upper thigh. Be careful not to arch or hyperextend your back. Repeat the stretch with your other leg.

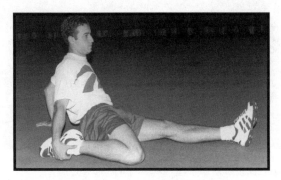

*Forward Lunge Stretch*

From a standing position step forward with your right leg with knee bent at 90 degrees. Place both hands on your thigh for support. Extend your left leg back with heel off of the floor. Repeat stretch with left leg bent and right leg extended back.

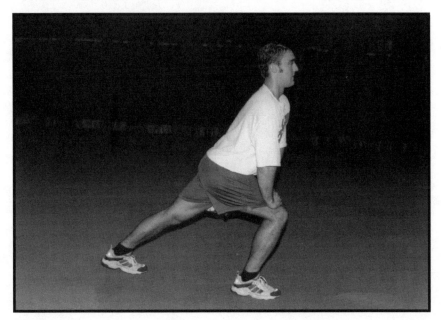

*Lying on Stomach Quad Stretch*

Lie on your stomach with legs extended behind you. Flex one leg at the knee and bring the heel towards your buttock. Reach back with your arm, grasp your ankle, and slowly pull the heel closer to your buttock until you feel tension in the thigh. Repeat the stretch with your opposite leg.

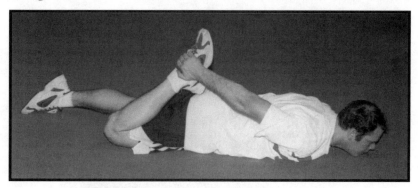

*Standing Quad Stretch*

Stand facing a wall at arms length. Use your right arm to brace yourself against the wall. Flex your right leg at the knee. Use your left arm to reach behind and grasp your right ankle. Slowly pull your heel toward your buttock until you feel a stretch in your upper thigh. Repeat stretch with opposite leg.

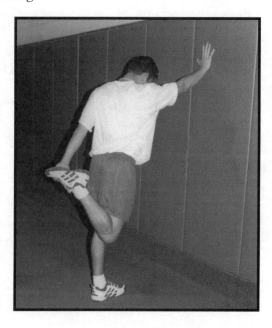

CALVES

### Partner Lean

Stand facing a partner at arms length. Position your feet several inches apart and parallel to each other. Lean forward with arms outstretched and hands braced against your partner's shoulders. Keep your feet and heels flat on the ground as you lean forward.

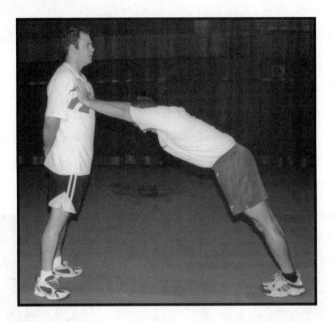

### Push-up Position Calf Stretch

Assume a push-up position. Place one foot on top of the heel of the opposite (balance) foot. Slowly push backward with your arms and try to lower the heel of the balance foot to the ground. Push as far as possible without pain. Repeat stretch with each leg.

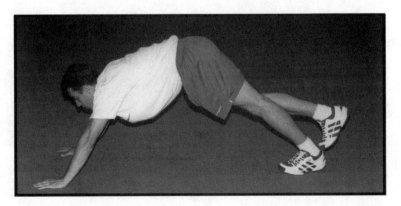

GROIN

### Sitting Groin Stretch

Assume a sitting position with the soles of your feet together in front of you. While holding your feet, place your elbows on the inside surface of your legs just above the knees. Use your elbows to gently push down on the inside of your knees.

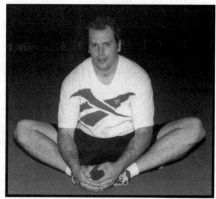

### Lying Groin Stretch

Lie flat on your back. Flex your knees and place the soles of your feet together in front of you. Spread your legs as far as you can as you try to lower the outside area of each knee as close to the ground as possible.

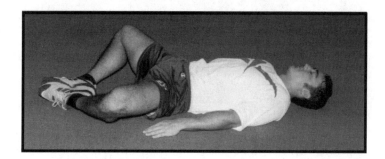

BACK

### Roll Ball Around Feet

Assume a sitting position with legs together and knees flexed. Slowly roll a soccer ball in a complete circle around your feet and your back. Try to keep both hands on the ball at all times. Complete five revolutions in one direction, then repeat for five revolutions in the opposite direction.

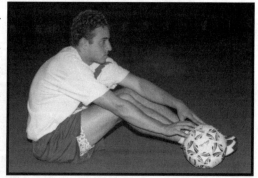

*Standing Lower Back Stretch*

Stand with feet spread apart, knees flexed, and a ball directly beneath you. Cross your arms, bend forward at the waist, and try to touch one elbow to the ball. Return to upright position and repeat stretch with opposite elbow.

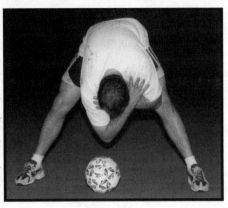

*Lying Back Stretch*

Lie on your back with arms extended to sides. Slowly bring your knees up toward your chin as far as possible without raising your arms and hands off the floor. Lift your hips slightly off the floor.

## NECK

*Head Turns*

Turn your head as far as possible toward the left. Hold that position, then turn your head to the right and repeat.

*Static Neck Stretch*

Place your right hand on the left side of your head. Slowly pull your head down and sideways toward your right shoulder. Do not jerk. Repeat stretch to opposite side.

## SHOULDERS

*Behind the Back Arm Stretch*

Extend both arms behind you with hands at approximately waist level. Interlock fingers and, while keeping arms straight, gradually raise arms to mid-back height. Hold stretch, relax, and repeat.

*Elbow Pull*

Place one arm behind your head with el-

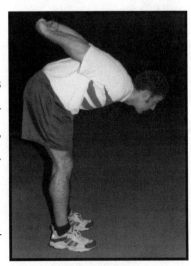

bow bent at 90 degrees. Grab the elbow with your opposite arm and hand and pull it further behind your head. Repeat stretch with opposite arm behind head.

### Arm Across Chest Stretch

Extend your left arm across the front of your chest. Grab the left elbow with your right hand and gently pull to the right to assist the stretch. Repeat stretch using left hand to stretch right arm across chest. *(photo on right)*

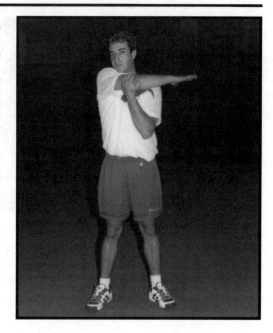

## Agility

Agility is a measure of your ability to change position and direction rapidly without loss of balance or speed. It is a critical element affecting soccer performance because players are required to constantly change speed and direction both with and without the ball. Agility depends upon a number of fitness components including strength, power, balance, speed, coordination and flexibility. Because agility in soccer is generally associated with specific skills, there isn't a single measure of agility that can be generalized to all situations. However, you can improve your overall level of agility through practice and game experience. It is also important to consider that agility will diminish with the onset of fatigue. Maintaining a high level of aerobic and muscular fitness will help you to maintain your agility over the course of a soccer match.

## AGILITY DRILLS

### Shuttle Run

Place two cones 20 yards apart (distance can vary) to represent side boundaries. Place a third cone midway between the two side boundaries. From the middle cone sprint to the boundary to your right, touch the ground with your hand, turn and sprint to the left boundary and touch the ground, turn and sprint to the middle.

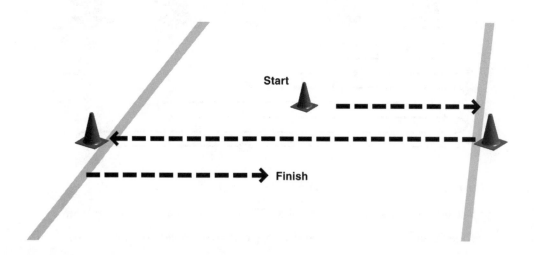

### Triangle Cone Agility Drill

This drill is designed to improve your ability to change direction without losing speed. Place three cones five yards apart in the shape of a triangle. Start at cone A. Sprint to cone B, turn and sprint to cone C, sprint back to cone B, then backpedal to cone C.

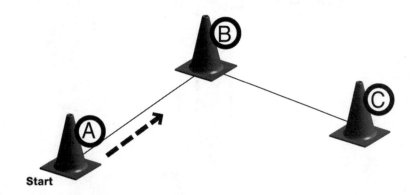

*Line Drill*

Place five cones in a straight line with 10 yards distance between adjacent cones. Start at cone A. Sprint to cone B, turn and sprint back to A. Immediately sprint to cone C, turn and sprint back to A, sprint to D, turn and sprint back to A, sprint to E, turn and sprint to A. You are finished. Total distance covered in one rep is 200 yards.

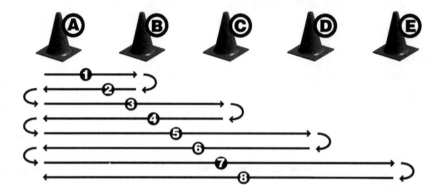

*T-Cone Drill*

Place four cones in the shape of a "T". Position cone B 10 yards from cone A, and place cones C and D 5 yards to each side of cone B. You position at cone A to begin. Sprint to cone B, side-shuffle left to cone C, immediately side-shuffle right to cone D, side-shuffle back to cone B, then back pedal to cone A. Total distance covered on one rep is 40 yards.

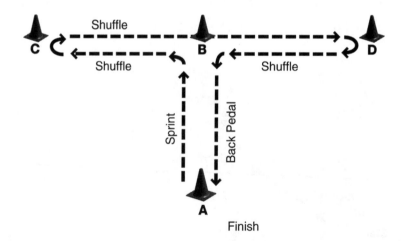

*Square Cone Run*

Place 4 cones 10 yards apart in the shape of a square. Start at cone A. Sprint to B, shuffle left to C, back pedal to D, then cariocca to cone A. Total distance covered in one rep is 40 yards.

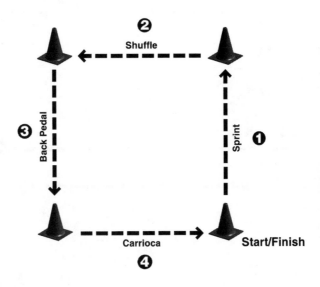

*Lateral Jumps*

Jump side-to-side with feet together over a 12-inch cone. Repeat as many jumps as possible in 30 seconds. (Time can vary, or you can perform the drill for a predetermined number of jumps).

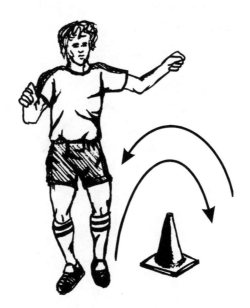

*Lateral Shuffle Movement*

Place two cones 12 feet apart. Side-shuffle laterally back and forth between cones. Do not cross your feet when shuffling. Six continuous repetitions equal one set.

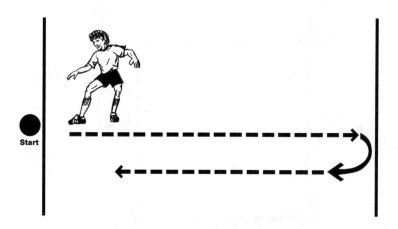

*Zig Zag Drill*

Place 10 cones in a zig zag formation with 10 yards distance between consecutive cones. Begin a cone #1. Sprint to #2, then #3, then #4 etc. until you have reached the end of the line of cones. Lower your center of gravity as you approach each cone, plant your outside foot, open your hips, and drive to the next cone.

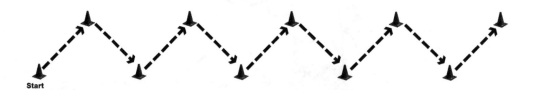

### Five Cone Box Drill

Position 4 cones in the shape of a square with 10 yards distance between cones. Place a cone in the center of the square. Starting from the center cone, sprint to cone A, sprint back to center, sprint to cone B, back to center, sprint to cone C, back to center, sprint to cone D, back to center. A completed circuit equals one rep.

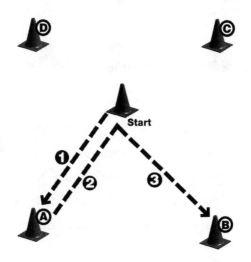

### Cone Chute Drill

Place 10 cones in a slalom-like course with 5 yards distance between cones. Beginning at the first cone, weave throughout the slalom course at maximum speed. One length of course equals one rep.

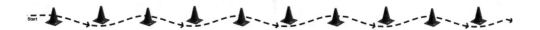

*Sprint/Shuffle/Sprint*

Place four cones in a straight line with 20 yards distance between cones. Starting at the cone #1, sprint to cone #2, rotate body sideways and shuffle to #3, as you reach cone #3 rotate body forward and sprint to cone #4. Total distance covered is 60 yards per repetition. Perform 10 reps at maximum speed with a 25 second rest between reps.

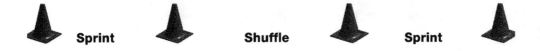

*Sprint/Shuffle Laterally/Sprint/Shuffle Laterally/Sprint*

Place 6 cones in a configuration as illustrated. Keep 15 yards distance between cones. Begin at cone #1. Sprint to #2, side-shuffle to #3, sprint to #4, side-shuffle to #5, sprint to #6. Sequence of six cones equals one rep. Perform 10 to 15 reps with a short rest between each repetition.

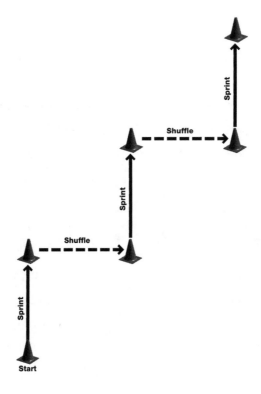

# 9 Plyometric Training

Plyometric – or jump – training became popular in Europe during the late 1970s. A form of dynamic action resistance training used to develop explosive power and jumping ability, plyometrics provide an overload to the musculature in a way that is somewhat different from weight training. In effect, plyometric training bridges the gap between strength and speed training by effectively combining elements of each to develop increased power and explosiveness.

Plyometric training enhances the ability of your muscles to respond more quickly and powerfully to changes in muscle length. Many movements in soccer, such as jumping to head a ball or suddenly changing speed and direction while dribbling, involve lengthening (eccentric) muscle contractions rapidly followed by shortening (concentric) contractions. The more quickly the concentric contraction follows the eccentric contraction, the greater the power generated. Plyometric training is designed to speed up the eccentric-concentric contraction phase which in turn enhances your ability for

Plyometric training enhances the ability of your muscles to respond more quickly and powerfully to changes in muscle length.

explosive-type movement.

Although plyometric training typically focuses on the development of lower body strength and power, in some instances it can also be used to develop arm speed and strength in sports like baseball and volleyball. Plyometrics are particularly effective for developing the explosive leg power needed for soccer. Most exercises involve rapid changes of direction such as hopping, jumping, skipping, or bounding, and place great demands on the muscles and connective tissues. To maximize the training effect and minimize the likelihood of injury, adhere to the following guidelines when performing plyometric exercises.

√ Perform plyometric exercises on a soft surface (preferably grass), and wear quality athletic shoes with plenty of ankle and arch support.

√ Weight training complements plyometric training. It is important to establish an adequate strength base prior to beginning a plyometric training program.

√ Perform plyometrics 2 or 3 days per week for 15 to 20 minutes per session. Excessive training and/or improper technique can lead to knee problems, so stop at the first sign of discomfort.

√ Perform each exercise in quality fashion. Emphasize height and/ or distance of each jump with minimal ground contact time. Treat the ground as it were hot coals and you were in bare feet - as soon as you contact ground begin your next jump.

## Plyometric Exercises

### Double-Leg Hop

Stand erect, shoulders facing forward, with arms at your sides. Begin by jumping up and flexing your legs to bring your heels to your buttocks.

Upon landing, immediately jump up again. Perform 15 to 20 jumps, rest, and repeat.

*Single-Leg Hop*

Similar to the double-leg hop except that all jumping is done on one leg. Hold the opposite leg in a flexed position as you jump. Perform 5 to 10 jumps with one leg, then repeat with the opposite leg. Perform 2 to 3 sets with each leg.

*Lateral Jumps*

Stand beside a 12-inch cone with feet together and toes pointing forward. Jump sideways back and forth over the cone for 30 seconds. Rest for one minute, then repeat.

*Skate Bounding*

This exercise simulates power ice skating on dry land. Push off with as much power as possible with each leg. Spend as much time in the air as possible as you jump from one leg to the other.

*Depth Jumps*

Stand on top of a box 18 to 24 inches high. Step off of the box, land on both feet, and explode upward as high as possible. Concentrate on springing upward at the instant your feet touch the ground.

*Bench Jump*

Stand approximately two feet in front of a bench 18 to 24 inches high. Swing your arms upward to generate momentum and jump up onto the bench. Land with your feet together. Immediately jump back to the ground and repeat the jump. Perform 10 to 15 jumps at maximum speed, rest, and then repeat.

*Bounding Over Distance*

With feet together, jump diagonally forward to the right, then to the left, then right, etc. Continue bounding forward over a distance of 20 yards, rest, and then repeat.

*Tuck Jump*

From an upright position lower your body by bending at the knees until your thighs are parallel to the ground. Keep your back straight and chest out. Explode upward and bring your knees to your chest while in the air. Repeat 8 to 10 times at maximum speed , rest, and then repeat.

*Sideways Hop for Distance*

Position 8 to 10 cones in a row with one yard distance between cones. Stand sideways to the first cone with feet together and toes straight ahead. Jump sideways over the first cone, then the second, then the third, and so on until you've reached the last cone. Rest, then repeat the sequence in the opposite direction.

*Power Skips*

Begin skipping forward in a normal fashion, then gradually progress to the power skip. Thrust the knee of your lead leg upward toward your chest. At the same time thrust your opposite arm upward. Continue skipping over a distance of 30 yards, bounding as high as you can with opposite arm and leg thrusting upward in unison.

*Rope Skipping*

Jump rope using single, double, and alternate leg fashion. Focus on continuous rebounding. React as soon as your feet contact the ground.

*Push-up Depth Jump (for upper body strength and power)*

Assume a push-up position. Slowly lower your body to the ground, then explode upward with your hands coming off of the ground. While off the ground spread your arms apart and land with hands in a wider push-up position. Repeat.

# 10 Eating for Peak Performance

What an athlete eats on a daily, weekly, and monthly basis can significantly affect his or her performance on the playing field. This is especially true in soccer where the energy demands are great and the body's ability to supply the working muscles with energy can become a limiting factor in performance. By eating the right foods before, during and after training and competition, soccer players can maximize their energy reserves and perform at peak efficiency for an entire game, a weekend tournament, and even an entire season. Before we go any further, however, it is important to realize that there are no magical foods that will transform average players into great players. Even the most nutritious diet will not compensate for shortcomings in fitness, skill, and tactical ability. All other things being equal, however, what you eat and when you eat it can be a factor in determining whether or not you play well, particularly in the later stages of a game.

## High Energy Diet

Most school and college-age athletes don't have the benefit of a carefully planned, nutritionally sound training table. They take their meals in a variety of places ranging from mom's kitchen to the drive-through window of the local fast food establishment. Even so, it is still relatively easy for soccer players to consume a healthy, high-energy diet. All that's needed is a bit of nutritional know-how coupled with intelligent food choices.

The energy used for muscular activity, commonly measured in units called calories, is derived primarily from the carbohydrates and fats in our diet. Proteins, although an important dietary staple, are not an energy source except in extreme situations. Their primary role in the body is to serve as the building blocks for growth and repair of cells. Nutritionists suggest that a well-balanced, high-energy diet should derive 60 to 65% of calories from carbohydrates, 20 to 25% of calories from fat, and 10 to 15% of calories from protein. The typical American diet, in contrast, gets nearly 40% of calories from fat, contains too much protein, and too little carbohydrate. From an energy and overall health standpoint, the typical American diet is not the best diet for soccer players. For that reason you must make a conscious effort to consume a diet that may be atypical of your friends and family, one that contains a greater percentage of complex carbohydrates along with lesser amounts of fat and protein.

**Carbohydrates** are the sugars and starches found in foods such as pasta, rice, vegetables, cereals, fruits, milk and milk products. Our body breaks down the carbohydrates that we eat and stores them in the form of a starch called glycogen. Some glycogen is stored in the liver, while the majority is stored in the muscles. When needed, glycogen can be readily broken down into molecules of glucose, or blood sugar, the primary fuel for our brain and muscle cells. Our body's glycogen stores are limited, and must be replaced on a regular basis. Gradual and chronic depletion of stored glycogen will decrease endurance and athletic performance.

**Fats** provide us with a highly concentrated source of food energy. One gram of fat contains approximately 9 calories of energy, compared to 4 calories per gram for both carbohydrates and protein. We obtain dietary fats primarily from meats, fish, dairy products, nuts and vegetable oils. Excess fat is stored in fat cells called adipose tissue, and also in the muscle cells. Both glycogen and stored fats are available for use whenever the body needs energy above and beyond that supplied by the blood sugar.

The exact mix of fuel used by your muscles depends upon how hard you are working. During light and moderate exercise, such as pre-game warm-up, muscles run on a mixture of free fatty acids and glucose. As the intensity of exercise increases fats become a less efficient energy source. Glycogen is actually the preferred fuel for both short-term (sprint) and long-term (endurance) exercise. During a soccer game your muscles must draw on stored glycogen for energy. As supplies run short your muscles will become exhausted and fail to perform properly. You can maximize muscle glycogen stores by increasing carbohydrate intake during the three or four days prior to a game. During the same period you should gradually reduce the intensity and volume of training.

The type of carbohydrate consumed is not particularly important with respect to energy storage. Both complex (starches) and simple (sugars) carbohydrates are effective in increasing glycogen stores. For general health reasons, however, it is better to eat a greater percentage of nutrient-dense, complex carbohydrates such as pasta, rice, vegetables, cereals, and grains as opposed to large quantities of sweets and simple sugars.

## Eating on the Road

Many soccer players don't have nutritionally sound meals prepared for them when commuting to and from games. Fast-food restaurants, noted for the high fat, salt, and sugar content of their foods, are often the site of pre- and post-game meals. Even so, by following a few simple guidelines you will find ample opportunity to consume healthy, high-energy meals at most any restaurant.

√ Choose complex carbohydrate foods such as cereals, pancakes, waffles, bagels, toast with honey or jelly, potatoes, pastas, rice and fruits. Go easy on items like doughnuts and pastries, which are generally high in fat and loaded with simple sugars.

√ Go light on fried foods such as eggs, bacon, cheese, and ham. They contain high concentrations of protein and fat, and are difficult to digest in a short amount of time.

√ Drink plenty of fruit juices. Natural juices are low in fat and high in carbohydrates.

√ Pizza, although relatively high in fat due to the cheese covering, is also a good carbohydrate source. Choose vegetable toppings (green peppers, onions, mushrooms) rather than high- fat meat toppings – and go easy on the cheese.

√ Eat plenty of bread and rolls, but skip the butter or margarine or use it sparingly.

√ If you must eat red meat, choose broiled or baked rather than fried. The same goes with fish.

√ Select baked or broiled potatoes rather than french fries.

√ Don't smother foods with creamy gravies or sauces; toppings are usually high in fat.

√ Drink skim or two-percent milk rather than whole milk.

√ At the salad bar eat all of the fresh vegetables that you want, but go easy on fried side-bar items (chicken wings, fried bread, fried mushrooms, etc.) and salad dressings. Items such as macaroni salad or pastas mixed with mayonnaise or similar fat-laden condiments should be taken sparingly. As a general rule, the plainer the food the better it is for you.

√ For dessert eat ice milk or sherbet. Although ice cream is a good source of carbohydrates, it also contains the highest concentration of fat. Gelatin is also a good dessert choice since it's low in fat and high in carbohydrates.

**KEY WORDS TO LOOK FOR ON RESTAURANT MENUS**

The following words indicate a high-fat food item, and are not good choices for the pre-game meal: fried, breaded, crispy, scampi style, creamed, buttery, au gratin, gravy. It is okay to eat higher-fat entrees for the post-game meal because you probably won't compete again within the next 24 hours. If you are scheduled to play sooner, however, it's best to stick with carbohydrates at the post-game meal as well.

## Pre- and Post-Game Nutrition

There are no special foods that, when taken several hours prior to a match, will guarantee a super performance. The greatest performance benefits will come from proper eating on a daily, weekly, and even monthly basis. Even so, what you eat and drink prior to a game can to some extent affect your performance.

### PRE-COMPETITION GUIDELINES

*Few Days Before*

When you have several days to nutritionally prepare for a game, begin to taper your training 2 or 3 days prior to the match. During that same period increase the percentage of carbohydrates in your diet. This process of carbohydrate restocking can continue up until a few hours before the game.

*Evening Before*

What you eat the evening before a game may actually be more important than what you eat the day of the game. Your overall nutritional goal is to properly hydrate your body and at the same time increase carbohydrate fuel stores. A suitable, high carbohydrate meal could include one or more of the following items: pasta with marinara sauce, baked potatoes with low-fat cheese and vegetables, small amounts of meat, rice, breads, fruits, ice milk or sherbet. Hydrate your body at regular intervals rather than in one sitting. Drink 4 to 8 extra glasses of fluid throughout the day prior to the game.

*Pre-Game Meal*

The primary goals of the pre-game meal are to : 1) provide energy to the muscles; 2) ward off feelings of hunger when competing; 3) ensure that you are well-hydrated; 4) prevent upset stomach during competition. The following guidelines will help you to accomplish those goals.

√ Consume the meal 3 to 4 hours before the game. This will provide sufficient time for the stomach and upper small intestine to empty prior to competition.

√ Carbohydrates should be the primary constituent of the pre-game meal. They are easily digested and will help to maintain blood glucose levels. Pancakes, waffles, bagels, muffins, toast and jelly, fruit, pasta, vegetables and rice are all good choices (but not at the same meal!).

√ Keep the meal low in fats and proteins because both of these nutrients are digested slowly. Nutritionists no longer advocate the traditional pre-game meal of steak and eggs.

√ Avoid greasy and highly seasoned foods

√ Don't experiment with different foods before a big game! Include familiar foods that you enjoy.

There will be times when you won't be able to consume the pre-game meal 3 to 4 hours prior to the match. This may occur when playing a series of games in a weekend tournament, or when the kickoff is scheduled early in the day. In such cases the timing of the pre-game meal will determine your food choices. Table 10.2 provides guidelines to assist you in making the best choices.

## Table 10.1
## SAMPLE PRE-GAME MEALS

| Meal #1 | Meal #2 |
|---|---|
| 1 cup oatmeal with fruit | 4 pancakes with syrup |
| 1 cup skim milk | 1 cup fruit cocktail |
| 1 English muffin with jelly | 1 cup skim milk |
| 8 oz sport drink | 8 oz orange juice |

## Table 10.2
## TIME FOOD CHOICES

| | |
|---|---|
| 3-4 hours before game | bread products, pasta, sandwiches, juices, fruit, yogurt, bagels, pancakes, waffles, baked potatoes |
| 2-3 hours before game | juices, fruit, yogurt, bread products, pancakes |
| 1 hour before game | fruit juice, fresh fruit, high carbohydrate beverage, English muffin with jelly |

### POST-COMPETITION GUIDELINES

Proper refueling after a game is also important, especially if you are going to play two or three matches over the span of several days. The following guidelines will help to offset fatigue and aid in the recovery process.

√ Drink plenty of fluids immediately following the game and throughout the remainder of the day to replace water and minerals lost through sweat.

√ Start glycogen replacement within an hour after the game by drinking diluted fruit juices or energy-replacement drinks.

√ Eat a large meal consisting primarily of complex carbohydrates (pasta, rice, potatoes, bread) approximately three hours after the game. A high carbohydrate meal serves to replenish depleted glycogen stores.

## Fluid Replacement

Inadequate hydration, even more so than diet, is a major cause of poor performance, fatigue, and illness. This is especially true when playing and training in hot, humid environments. Performance is usually impaired when water loss exceeds 3 percent of body weight, as is the ability to effectively regulate body heat. You should replenish fluids at regular intervals during training sessions and games, whether you feel thirsty or not. Thirst is not an accurate indicator of fluid needs. In fact, you usually won't experience a feeling of thirst until you've already suffered a water loss

| Table 10.3 COMMERCIALLY AVAILABLE FLUID SUPPLEMENT SPORT DRINKS (8 oz. serving) | | |
|---|---|---|
| Brand | Calories | Carbohydrates (gm) |
| All Sport | 70 | 19 |
| Break Through | 80 | 20 |
| CytoMax | 80 | 16 |
| Endura | 60 | 15 |
| Exceed | 70 | 17 |
| Gatorade | 50 | 14 |
| Mountain Dew Sport | 95 | 16 |
| Powerade | 70 | 19 |
| Power Surge | 75 | 18 |
| 10-K | 60 | 15 |
| Winner's Edge | 75 | 18 |

of 1% of body weight. In addition, feelings of thirst can be satisfied well before you have consumed enough fluids to replace that which was lost through perspiration.

You should start monitoring your fluid intake two or three days prior to the game. Consume foods that contain a high water content , such as fruits and vegetables, and drink plenty of fluids. On the day of competition take small quantities of fluid at regular intervals prior to and during the game. Water is always a good choice, and some of the commercial sport drinks also work well. When choosing sport drinks, pick ones that:

√ Contain few solid particles (low in sugar and salt content), and don't taste overly sweet.

√ Contain small amounts of the simple sugars glucose and sucrose to provide quick energy to the working muscles. The carbohydrate concentration should be sufficient to supply energy to the muscles without slowing absorption from the stomach.

√ Taste good. An appealing taste will encourage consumption.

## What to Drink and When to Drink It

### Before Game/Practice

Water, low-sugar sport drinks, tea and diet sodas without caffeine (if the carbonation doesn't bother you) are possible pregame choices. Ice tea is also a good bet on hot days, although the caffeine in tea is a diuretic so too much tea before or during competition isn't recommended. Fluids high in sugar content, such as regular soda pop and fruit juices, are fine for after the game but should be avoided immediately prior to and during the game. The high sugar content slows fluid absorption from the stomach.

### During Game/Practice

Some carbohydrate is okay, but too much is not good because it slows absorption from the stomach to the intestine. A concentration between 5 and 10% is recommended. Water, low-sugar sport drinks like Gatorade and All-Sport, and iced tea with a minimal amount of sugar are good choices. Drink frequently in small amounts. Aim for 3 to 6 ounces every 10 or 15 minutes. Regular soda is not a good choice during exercise. The sugar content is too high, the carbonation may make you feel uncomfortable, and the caffeine in most colas is a diuretic which makes you urinate and promotes water loss.

### After Game/Practice

Water, diluted fruit juices, soda, and sport drinks (See Table 10.3) are all fine. Sugary drinks are okay after the game because they help to replenish depleted energy stores.

## Vitamin and Mineral Supplements

Vitamins and minerals, commonly referred to as the micronutrients, are at the center of more myth and public ignorance than any single element of nutrition. Vitamins are classified as either fat soluble or water soluble. The fat soluble vitamins A, D, E, and K can be stored in the body, primarily in the liver and in fatty tissue. Because our body can store excesses of these vitamins we do not have to consume them every day. The water soluble vitamins (B complex and C) have little or no body storage, and must be replenished on a regular basis. Minerals are inorganic compounds found in trace amounts in the body. Most occur naturally in a variety of foods, and are categorized as either major or trace minerals (elements) according to their contribution to overall health.

Vitamins and minerals function primarily in the body's biochemical reactions, and do not provide fuel for energy metabolism. Both are needed in very small quantities. With regard to exercise, there does not appear to be an excessive demand for most vitamins and minerals during periods of increased activity. So, as a general rule, supplementing your diet with large amounts of vitamins and minerals above and beyond the minimum daily requirement is not warranted and will not improve physical performance. Most athletes can achieve their daily vitamin and mineral requirements through a normal, varied diet. If your diet is deficient, however, or if you have special needs, then supplementation may be warranted.

## Salt and Electrolyte Replacement

Your body depends on water and electrolytes (sodium, potassium, chloride) to regulate the transport of water into and out of cells. An electrolyte imbalance can cause cells to become dehydrated and ultimately leads to diminished performance. Because electrolytes are lost in sweat, replacement is always a concern. Most of the popular sport drinks on the market today are good sources of electrolytes, as are fruits and fruit juices.

In the past coaches and trainers often advocated the use of salt tablets to replace the sodium lost in sweat. This is not a good practice! Although it is true that some salt is lost in perspiration, the concentration of salt loss is not nearly as great as the concentration of water loss. Ingesting salt tablets distorts the desirable ratio of salt to water in the body. Concentrated doses of sodium also promote the loss of potassium, a mineral essential for the proper functioning of muscle cells. The best way to replace the salt lost in sweat is by lightly salting your meals. Most of us consume too much salt to begin with, a by-product of our typical American diet.

## Food for Thought

Proper nutrition is only one aspect affecting your performance on the soccer field. Although the guidelines suggested here are all supported by research, keep in mind that soccer players are individuals with their own ideas, beliefs, and food preferences. Many players are also superstitious, at least to a degree, and have favorite foods or food rituals which they believe help them to play better. Soccer players should not be forced to eat so called "proper" foods if they don't enjoy them, or don't believe that they are good for them. During my years as a professional player I observed some of the best players eating some of the worst meals you could imagine, at least from a nutritional standpoint. They still played very well, although they may have played even better if they watched their diet. We will never know. In any event, if push comes to shove, athletes should be allowed to eat foods that they believe will help them perform at their best, so long as they have eaten the foods before without gastrointestinal mishaps. In some cases the psychological benefits of eating what you "want" may outweigh the nutritional benefits of eating what you "should!"

# 11 Achieving Optimal Weight

In sports such as wrestling and horse racing athletes must make weight. This means that, to compete, they must keep their total body weight within a specified range. Although soccer players aren't required by the Laws of the Game to "make weight," they should maintain a weight that will enable them to compete at an optimal level of performance. Studies of endurance athletes competing in various sports strongly suggest that a high percentage of body fat is associated with diminished performance. Speed, endurance, balance, agility and jumping ability are all negatively affected by a high level of fatness.

The incomparable Pele, possibly the greatest player of all time, was of medium height and compactly built. Former Dutch star Johann Cruyff, considered by some to be the European equivalent of Pele, was thin almost to the degree of being considered "skinny." The moral of this story is that good soccer players come in all shapes and sizes. For that reason weight standards for soccer should be based on body composition, or ratio of fat to muscle, and not on how much a player actually weighs in pounds. Body weight is comprised of two primary components: body fat and fat-free (lean body ) tissue . When the weight of body fat is subtracted from total body weight, the remaining value is

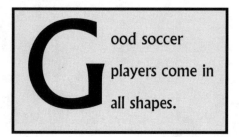

considered to be fat-free tissue. Fat-free tissue is comprised of skeletal muscle mass, organs, bones and skin. Muscle usually makes up about 50% of the fat-free tissue. Fat-free weight is considered to be positively correlated with athletic performance because a greater percentage of muscle translates to a greater potential for strength and power. The average adult male (non-athlete) averages between 12% and 15% body fat while females average somewhat higher between 18% and 23% body fat. Physically fit endurance athletes are substantially leaner. The optimal range for male soccer players is between 6 and 14% body fat, females between 12% and 18%. If a soccer player's percentage of body fat falls above or below the optimal range, performance will usually suffer.

## Assessing Body Composition

Estimates of body composition can be determined quickly and with a relatively high degree of accuracy. The most widely used field technique involves measuring skinfold fat thickness at several sites, and then using those measurement to estimate the percentage of total body fat. Measurements are taken at the triceps, scapula, and abdomen with an instrument called a skinfold caliper. The values are then plugged into a formula to determine the approximate percentage of fat and fat-free weight. An experienced trainer or coach using skin calipers can usually calculate percent body fat within an error range of 1 to 2 percent. Another method of calculating body composition involves underwater weighing. This technique provides even greater accuracy than skin calipers. The downside is that underwater weighing must be performed in a lab setting and is also more time consuming.

Once body composition has been determined, the amount of fat-free weight can be used to calculate what the athlete should weigh at a specific percent body fat. Table 11.1 illustrates the situation of a 150 pound male soccer player with 20%

body fat whose goal is to reduce to 12% body fat. We know that, at his goal weight, the player's body weight will consist of 12% fat and 88% lean body tissue. To estimate his goal weight at 12% fat we divide fat-free weight by 88%, the fraction of the player's goal weight that is to be represented by fat-free weight. This calculation provides a goal weight of 136 pounds. This player must lose 14 pounds of body fat while maintaining his present amount of fat-free weight to reach 12% body fat.

> **Table 11.1**
> **Determining Goal Weight for Male Soccer Player**
>
> Weight – 150 lbs.
>
> % Body fat – 20%
>
> Fat weight – 150 X 0.20 = 30 lbs.
>
> Fat-free weight –
>
> 150 lb. - 30 lbs. fat weight = 120 lb.
>
> Goal (% fat) –
>
> 12% = (88% fat-free weight)
>
> Goal weight – (120 lb./.88) = 136 lbs.
>
> **Weight loss goal 14 pounds**

The key element to consider in the above weight-loss scenario is the type of tissue lost. It is important that weight loss result from fat tissue loss, not muscle tissue loss. As we've discussed , loss of muscle tissue leads to diminished strength, stamina, and power. Your weight loss goal should always be to drop the weight without negatively impacting performance. .

## Guidelines for Losing Fat

Accumulating fat is our body's way of saving for a rainy day. One pound of body fat is equivalent to approximately 3500 calories of stored energy. If you are presently carrying a few extra pounds it is because, over time, you have consumed more calories than you needed to fuel daily activities. This is not an uncommon situation for athletes, particularly during the off-season when players are not as physically active. Accumulation of these "extra calories" usually occurs slowly over a period of weeks or even months. Fat deposition is an additive process with a flexible time frame. For example, if your caloric intake stays about the same during the off-season but you burn just 100 fewer calories per day, the equivalent of approximately 10 minutes of aerobic activity, over a period of four months you will gain approximately 5 pounds of fat.

The only proven way to lose fat is to burn up through everyday activities more calories than you consume, a situation commonly referred to as a caloric deficit.

When you create a deficit of 3500 calories, whether it be over a week, two weeks, or a month, you will lose one pound of fat. Double the deficit and you will double the fat loss. You can create a caloric deficit by eating less, exercising more, or a combination of both. Crash dieting, in and of itself, is not the answer. Severe dietary restriction results in loss of both muscle tissue and fat tissue. To compound the problem, crash diets typically require a major reduction in carbohydrate intake. You recall that carbohydrates are the primary energy source for endurance athletes. Insufficient carbohydrate intake depletes the body's glycogen stores, and makes it difficult to train or compete at a high level of intensity. Finally, because water storage accompanies carbohydrate storage, water stores are also diminished which further impairs the quality of training. In short, dieting doesn't work!

The most sensible approach to reducing body fat is to combine moderate caloric restriction with an increased volume of exercise. You can cut calories from your diet without giving up your favorite foods. Merely eliminate unnecessary fat calories. For example, eating a baked potato instead of mashed potatoes cuts fat and calories. The same goes when switching from whole to two-percent milk. There are myriad ways to cut hundreds of fat calories from your meals without substantially changing the quantity or quality of the foods eaten. While you are reducing the number of calories consumed each day, you can also burn additional calories by increasing the quantity of your training. The synergistic effect of fewer calories and more exercise will eventually lead to the desired result - fat loss. For example, creating a caloric deficit of 500 calories per day through modifications of eating and activity habits will result in a fat loss of approximately one pound per week. Actual weight loss in pounds may be more or less, depending upon water loss and/or retention and related factors. Your body weight may even increase if, during the same period of time you are losing fat, you are adding muscle to your frame through strength training.

In summary, to reduce body fat in a safe and effective manner you should:

√ Create a caloric deficit of approximately 3500 calories for each pound of body fat that you wish to lose.

√ Combine moderate dietary restriction with increased exercise.

√ Aim for a fat loss of 1 to 2 pounds per week. A caloric deficit of 500 to 1000 calories per day will achieve that goal. If you are losing weight at a faster rate it is probably due to losses in fat-free weight as well as body fat.

√ Don's skip meals. Caloric intake should be spread over a minimum of three meals consumed at regular intervals throughout the day.

√ An active athlete should not drop below 2000 calories per day to avoid vitamin and mineral deficiencies.

## Guidelines for Gaining or Maintaining Fat-Free Weight

At some point your goal may be to gain, or at least maintain, body weight. For the average person that sounds like a great problem to have because gaining weight is easy for most of us. For a soccer player, however, maintaining optimal body weight can sometimes be a real problem. This situation can occur during the course of a long, rigorous playing season, a period of time when you are expending a great amount of energy and effort each day. The simple solution would seem to be to consume more calories. Sorry to say, it's not that simple. Granted, taking in more calories than you need will undoubtedly result in weight gain. Unfortunately, the type of weight gained is body fat, and that is not what you want to do. Weight gains should reflect increases in fat-free weight. You recall that fat-free weight is positively associated with athletic performance. Adding muscle to your frame increases your strength, power, and explosive movement capability. Increases in body fat only serve to slow you down, and will ultimately diminish your performance on the soccer field.

Take into account the following guidelines when trying to gain fat-free weight. First, you must create a positive caloric balance; in other words, you must take in more calories than you expend. An excess of 2500 calories is required to gain one pound of muscle. This amount should not be taken in one day, but rather in small increments over a number of days. In addition to your regular meals, consume one or two smaller meals or snacks each day. The recommended daily caloric intake should not exceed expenditure by more than 1000 calories, however, which translates into a weight gain of approximately two pounds per week. Second, to ensure that the extra calories are laid down as muscle and not as fat, you must undertake a vigorous weight training program during the high calorie diet period. This is best

## Table 11.2
## LOW-FAT FOOD CHOICES
### (Less than 20% Calories from Fat)

**Produce**

Fruits and vegetables, dried fruit

**Starches**

Most breads and cereals, bagels, pasta, noodles, rice, corn, potatoes, pretzels, graham crackers

**Dairy Products**

Nonfat milk, 1% milk, buttermilk, low-fat yogurt, low-fat cottage cheese, ice milk , sherbet

**Protein Foods**

Most fish and seafood, chicken breast (without skin), egg whites, legumes, Canadian bacon

**Sugar Foods & Desserts**

Jam, jelly, fruit bars, apple butter, angel food cake, Jell-O, fig bars, low-fat frozen yogurt, popsicles

accomplished through heavy resistance, low repetition weight training that results in muscular hypertrophy.

Note: The extra calories consumed when attempting to gain fat-free weight should come from quality, nutrient rich foods. Complex carbohydrates like grains, cereals, and vegetables are recommended along with low-fat protein sources like chicken and fish. Don't add calories to your diet merely by consuming large quantities of high-fat, high-sugar, low-nutrient "junk foods." As the saying goes, "quality in, quality out."

# 12 Year-Round Training Program

By this point of the book you realize that conditioning is not merely a seasonal concern. The development and maintenance of peak soccer fitness requires year-round commitment and effort. Your goal is to achieve a high level of total body fitness prior to the beginning of the playing season. The best way to accomplish that is to approach fitness training from a long-term perspective. Plan your training around three general periods of time: off-season, preseason, and in-season.

## Endurance Training

The bulk of aerobic conditioning should take place during the off-season. Although it is possible to make significant improvements in aerobic fitness in as little as two or three months, it is safer and more effective if done over a longer time period. It is also important for you to develop a solid aerobic base before attempting more rigor-

**Table 12.1**
**ENDURANCE TRAINING:**
Seasonal Goals and Methods

**Off-Season**

**Fitness Goals:** Develop high level of general endurance. Quantity (aerobic) training designed to train slow twitch muscle fibers and improve cardiorespiratory endurance base.

**Methods:** Distance running, fartlek, interval training, soccer-specific exercises using the ball.

**Pre-Season**

**Fitness Goals:** Maintain solid aerobic fitness base. Increase anaerobic threshold through the use of "quality," high intensity training. The focus of preseason conditioning should be to sharpen skills and develop game-specific fitness.

**Methods:** Include more game-related drills in fitness training. Interval workouts with the ball can improve fitness and at the same time sharpen skills. Use longer work intervals (2 to 5 minutes); do not allow full recovery between work bouts.

**In-Season**

**Fitness Goals:** Maintain optimal levels of aerobic and anaerobic fitness. Train for soccer-specific speed.

**Methods:** Reduce training volume; focus on quality (anaerobic) training and speed training. Shorter work intervals (30 to 60 seconds) at maximum intensity. Functional (specific to playing position) and pressure training drills should comprise the majority of in-season drills. Less time devoted to fitness training without the ball.

ous, high intensity training at or near your anaerobic threshold. Use the interval training format to improve both aerobic and anaerobic fitness. Longer work intervals (3 to 5 minutes) focus more on the aerobic end of the continuum, while shorter, more intense work intervals (30 to 90 seconds) train the anaerobic energy pathways. Gradually include greater amounts of anaerobic (quality) training in your workouts as you near the playing season.

Once the season begins fitness training should focus entirely on high quality anaerobic work and speed training. Keep in mind that it doesn't take as much effort to maintain a high level of fitness as it does to develop it. Playing one or two games per week coupled with normal training between games will be sufficient to maintain levels of aerobic and anaerobic fitness during the season.

## Muscular Fitness Training

The greatest improvements in muscular fitness should also take place during the off-season. This is the time of the year when you have the opportunity to commit the greatest time and effort to developing total body strength.

## Table 12.2
## MUSCULAR FITNESS TRAINING
### Seasonal Goals and Methods

### Off-Season

**Fitness Goals:** Develop overall strength, flexibility and agility.
**Methods:** Commit to a total body workout designed to improve strength and muscular balance. Make use of the "progressive overload" principle to generate continued strength gains. Flexibility and agility training should also occur on a regular basis.

### Pre-Season

**Fitness Goals:** Emphasis gradually shifts from general strength training to training for power and muscular endurance. Incorporate plyometric exercises and sport-specific movements into your workout regimen.
**Methods:** Split your muscular fitness workouts between the weight room and the practice field. For example, to develop leg power jump side-to-side over a ball with feet together as rapidly as possible for 30 seconds, rest for 30 seconds, and then repeat. This type of plyometric-anaerobic interval training achieves two purposes - the development of power and improvement of anaerobic endurance.

### In-Season

**Fitness Goals:** Emphasis on power and speed of movement; maintenance of previous gains in muscular strength and endurance.
**Methods:** High-intensity training with the ball. Practice soccer skills and tactics at game speed and intensity. One or two maintenance strength workouts per week, coupled with normal training and game competition, will retain the muscular strength and power gains achieved prior to the season.

## Sample Off-season Conditioning Program

The following program was designed for college-age soccer players by Gary Wateska, strength and conditioning coach for Olympic Sports at the University of Pittsburgh. Gary's program utilizes various forms of distance running, sprint training, plyometrics, and agility drills, and covers an off-season period of approximately four months. You should notice that quantity training dominates the first several weeks of the program. Distance running and fartlek serve to improve aerobic capacity, and are also effective for maintaining, or lowering if need be, a player's level of body fat. As the program nears the start of the competitive season a greater portion of time is spent in quality, high-intensity, training. Sprint training is used to improve absolute speed and elevate the anaerobic threshold. Agility drills are added to improve overall quickness , reaction time, and ability to make sudden changes of speed and direction. Plyometric exercises are included to develop power and explosive movement.

Conditioning is scheduled on a Monday-Wednesday-Friday cycle. Strength training exercises (see Chapters 5 & 6), which are not listed in the following program, should be performed on a Tuesday-Thursday-Saturday cycle. Take off one day of training per week to rest, recuperate, and to stay mentally and physically fresh.

### POINTS TO KEEP IN MIND

1. Descriptions and illustrations of the agility drills listed in the program can be found in Chapter 8.

2. The program is designed for Division I college-age athletes, and is provided only as an example. In planning your individual program take into account your present state of fitness coupled with long-term goals and objectives.

3. In addition to a structured fitness program, you should play soccer and soccer-related training games as often as possible.

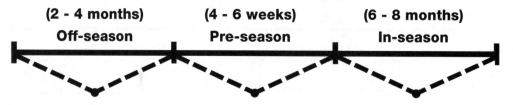

**(2 - 4 months)**  
**Off-season**

**(4 - 6 weeks)**  
**Pre-season**

**(6 - 8 months)**  
**In-season**

Off-season training emphasizes development of aerobic fitness, muscular strength, flexibility and agility. Training may include running, bicycling, fartlek, weight training, and flexibility exercises.

Pre-season training emphasizes development of match-related fitness. Drills should include a ball whenever possible. Interval training format is preferred option.

Technical and tactical training comprises the bulk of in-season training. Interval, pressure, and functional training are preferred during the season. Flexibility and agility must be maintained.

## WEEKLY TRAINING SCHEDULE

| Week #1 |
|---|
| **MONDAY** | ♦ 4 mile jog under 35 minutes<br>♦ 15 minutes of stadium running up and down stadium steps; run up, walk down<br>♦ 5 minutes of jump rope |
| **WEDNESDAY** | ♦ 1 mile jog<br>♦ 4 X 400 meter run under 1:40 minutes<br>♦ 6 X 200 meter run under 40 seconds ($^1/_2$ lap of quarter-mile track = 200 meters) |
| **FRIDAY** | ♦ 5 mile run (record your time) |

| Week #2 |
|---|
| **MONDAY** | ♦ Fartlek training on track: sprint the straight-aways, jog the curves for 2 miles<br>♦ Hill running: sprint to top of hill (40-50 yard sprint); walk down. repeat 10 times<br>♦ Agility drill: sprint/shuffle/sprint over 50 yards (using 10 yard sequences) |
| **WEDNESDAY** | ♦ 2 mile run under 12:30 minutes<br>♦ 5 X 100 yard sprints<br>♦ 10 X 40 yard sprints |
| **FRIDAY** | ♦ 30 minute jog<br>♦ 10 gassers (sprint across and back width of soccer field) - work:rest ratio 1:3 |

| Week #3 | |
| --- | --- |
| MONDAY | ◆ 10 X 100 yard acceleration sprints (30 yards at $^1/_2$ speed, 30 yards at $^3/_4$ speed, 40 yards at full speed) - work:rest ratio 1:1<br>◆ Agility drill: Sprint/Shuffle/Sprint: use 10 yard sequences over 50 yards (sprint 10 yards - shuffle laterally right 10 yards - sprint 10 yards - shuffle left 10 yards - sprint 10 yards; repeat 5 times<br>◆ 1 mile jog. |
| WEDNESDAY | ◆ 2 mile run under 12:30 minutes<br>◆ Stadium step runs (15 repetitions - run up, walk down) |
| FRIDAY | ◆ 4 mile jog<br>◆ Agility drills:<br>　1. zig zag drill over 25 yards (10 reps)<br>　2. shuffle-turn-sprint over 20 yards (shuffle laterally 10 yards, turn and sprint 10 yards)<br>　3. five cone drill using a 20 yard square box |

| Week #4 | |
| --- | --- |
| MONDAY | ◆ 1 mile jog<br>◆ 2 X 400 meter sprints under 1:30 minutes<br>◆ 2 X 200 meter sprints under 35 seconds<br>◆ 4 X 100 meter sprints under 20 seconds<br>◆ 8 X 80 yard sprints (maximum speed) — work:rest ratio 1:2 |
| WEDNESDAY | ◆ Five minute run/rest cycle: run 5 minutes - rest 5 minutes- run 5 minutes-rest 5 minutes-run 5 minutes — each 5 minute run should be longer than the previous run<br>◆ Agilities:<br>　1. carrioca 5 X 30 yards<br>　2. carrioca 15 yards-turn-sprint 15 yards (5 repetitions)<br>　3. shuttle run with 30 yard boundaries (10 repetitions)<br>◆ Plyometrics:<br>　1. lateral jumps over line (3 X 45 seconds)<br>　2. front/back jumps over line (3 X 20 seconds)<br>　3. tuck jumps (3 sets of 10) |
| FRIDAY | ◆ 3 mile jog<br>◆ 10 X 100 yard sprints (all-out effort on each sprint) — work:rest ratio 1:2 |

| Week #5 | |
|---|---|
| **MONDAY** | ♦ Jog 1.5 miles<br>♦ Ten 120 yard acceleration sprints (first 30 yards ½ speed, middle 30 yards ¾ speed, final 60 yards full speed<br>♦ Plyometrics:<br>   1. lateral cone hops (3 X 40 seconds)<br>   2. cone hops covering distance (10 cones) - perform 10 repetitions with rest between each rep.<br>   3. jump rope: speed jumping for one minute (3 reps with rest between) — work:rest ratio 1:1 |
| **WEDNESDAY** | ♦ 3 mile run under 22 minutes<br>♦ 10 X 50 yard sprints<br>♦ 5 X 40 yard sprint — work:rest ratio 1:2 |
| **FRIDAY** | ♦ 20 minutes of aerobic work with the ball<br>♦ Agilities:<br>   1. sprint/shuffle/sprint over 50 yards (10 reps)<br>   2. t-cone drill (5 reps)<br>   3. five cone box drill X 5 |

Once the season begins fitness training should focus entirely on high-quality anaerobic work and speed training.

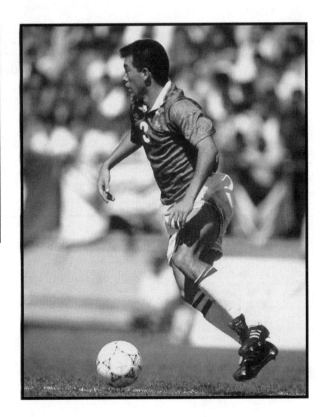

| Week #6 | |
|---|---|
| **MONDAY** | ♦ 3 mile jog<br>♦ Agility drills:<br>   1. cone chute over 50 yards X 10<br>   2. lateral jump over soccer ball (3 X 30 seconds)<br>   3. front/back jump over ball (3 X 20 seconds)<br>♦ Plyometrics:<br>   1. quick leaps (3 X 30 seconds)<br>   2. cone hops covering distance (5 X 20 yards) |
| **WEDNESDAY** | ♦ Hollow sprints - sprint 50 yards; jog 50 yards; walk 50 yards = one cycle (repeat 10 X)<br>♦ Full gassers - sprint across and back the width of soccer field (10 reps) - work:rest ratio 1:2<br>♦ Agility drills:<br>   1. sprint/shuffle/sprint X 10 (sprint 20 yd./shuffle 20 yd./sprint 20 yd. = 1 rep)<br>   2. triangle cone X 10 reps<br>♦ Plyometrics:<br>   1. box jumps (3 X 10)<br>   2. quick leaps (3 X 30 seconds)<br>   3. lateral movement over box, keeping one foot on box at all times (3 X 30 seconds) |
| **FRIDAY** | ♦ 30 minutes of aerobic work with the ball<br>♦ Plyometrics:<br>   1. tuck jumps (3 X 10)<br>   2. long jumps (3 X 30 yards)<br>   3. quick leaps (3 X 30 seconds)<br>♦ Agility drills:<br>   1. zig zag X 10 (over 20 yards)<br>   2. cone chute drill (over 40 yards) X 10 |

| Week #7 |  |
|---|---|
| MONDAY | ◆ 3 X 5 minute run (run 5/walk 5/run 5/walk 5/ run 5 – each 5 minute run farther than the previous one)<br>◆ Run up stadium steps/walk down (15 minutes)<br>◆ Agilities:<br>  1. sprint/shuffle/sprint/shuffle/sprint over 25 yards using 5 yard increments<br>  2. triangle cone drill X 5<br>  3. square cone drill X 10 |
| WEDNESDAY | ◆ Sprints: 4 X 400 meters; 2 X 200 meters; 1 X 800 meters<br>◆ Agilities:<br>  1. shuttle run using 30-yard boundaries X 5<br>  2. triangle cone drill X 5<br>  3. jump rope - speed jump for one minute/rest/repeat (5 reps) — work:rest ratio 1:1<br>◆ Plyometrics:<br>  1. free jumps (3 X 10)<br>  2. lateral cone hops covering distance (3 X 10 cones) |
| FRIDAY | ◆ 2 mile run (under 13 minutes)<br>◆ Shuttle runs over 30 yards (sprint 10 yards and back to start, 20 and back, 30 and back) for total of 120 yards each rep; perform 6 reps — Work:rest ratio 1:2 |

| Week #8 |  |
|---|---|
| MONDAY<br>&<br>FRIDAY | ◆ 15 X 100 yard sprints (first 5 at $\frac{1}{2}$ speed; second 5 at $\frac{3}{4}$ speed, last 5 at full speed) - work:rest ratio — 1:3<br>◆ Agility drills:<br>  1. sprint 10 yards; shuffle right 10 yards; back-pedal 5 yards; sprint diagonal 5 yards; shuffle right 5 yards; sprint 20 yards; perform 5 repetitions with rest in-between |
| WEDNESDAY | ◆ Jog 4 miles under 35 minutes |

## Week #9

| MONDAY | ◆ Sprint training: 10 sprints X 100 yards (full recovery between sprints)<br>◆ Aerobic/anaerobic training: 10 sprints X 60 yards (sprint 60 yards; slow jog back to start; repeat)<br>◆ Plyometrics:<br>  1. box jumps (3 X 10)<br>  2. single leg depth jumps (3 X 10)<br>  3. four line hops (3 X 30 seconds) |
|---|---|
| WEDNESDAY | ◆ 2 mile run under 12 minutes 20 seconds<br>◆ Hill running X 10 reps (50 yard uphill sprints)<br>◆ Agility drills:<br>  1. cone chute 4 X 60 yards — cones staggered every 10 yards<br>  2. five cone box drill X 10<br>  3. zig zag sprint drill - position cones every 5 yards in zig zag formation over 60 yards (complete 6 repetitions with rest in-between) |
| FRIDAY | ◆ 300 yard shuttle run X 4 repetitions (2 minute rest between repetitions)<br>◆ Stadium step running for 20 minutes (run up steps, slow jog down) |

## Week #10

| MONDAY | ◆ Down and back sprints: 1 X 100 yards ( sprint 100 yards, turn, sprint back = 1 rep) Reps = 1 X 90; 1 X 80; 1 X 70; 1 X 60; 1 X 50; 1 X 40; 1 X 100 — work:rest ratio 1:2<br>◆ Plyometrics:<br>  1. tuck jumps (cover distance 4 X 30 yards)<br>  2. bounding (cover distance 4 X 20 yards)<br>  3. lateral jumps over cone (3 X 30 seconds)<br>  4. jump rope 5 minutes |
|---|---|
| WEDNESDAY | ◆ 30 yard hollow sprints X 10 (Sprint 30 yards, jog 30 yards, walk 30 yards = 1 rep)<br>◆ Half gassers X 10 (half gasser = sprint width of soccer field)<br>◆ Agility drills:<br>  1. t-cone drill X 10<br>  2. zig zag drill X 5 reps (cover 20 yards, make minimum of 8 cuts)<br>  3. shuttle run using 20 yard boundaries X 5 reps<br>  4. sprint/shuffle/sprint over 40 yards X 10 reps |
| FRIDAY | ◆ 45 minutes of aerobic work (stairmaster, bike, jog) |

| Week #11 |  |
|---|---|
| **MONDAY** | ♦ Fartlek training X 20 minutes (use quarter mile track - sprint straight-aways, jog curves)<br>♦ Plyometrics:<br>  1. Tuck jumps with heel kick (3 sets/10 reps)<br>  2. standing long jump (3 set over 20 yard distance)<br>  3. jump rope:<br>    3 X 1:00 minute max speed<br>    3 X 1:00 minute double jump every other rotation<br>    3 X 20 yard distance while jumping rope |
| **WEDNESDAY** | ♦ 2 X 1 mile run (record time) - rest 10 minutes between mile runs<br>♦ Agility drills:<br>  1. shuffle/sprint/shuffle over 30 yards (10 reps)<br>  2. lateral movement (5 reps X 30 seconds/rep)<br>  3. five cone box drill (5 reps)<br>  4. twenty yard shuttle run (3 reps) |
| **FRIDAY** | ♦ 10 X 100 yard sprints (all sprints at max speed) – work:rest ratio – 1:3<br>♦ 10 X 60 yard sprints - work:rest ratio 1:2<br>♦ 10 X 40 yard sprints - work:rest ratio 1:2 |

| Week #12 |  |
|---|---|
| **MONDAY & FRIDAY** | ♦ Fartlek training - 1.5 miles<br>♦ Plyometrics:<br>  1. jump rope 1 minute at max speed (5 reps)<br>  2. tuck jumps (3 sets/10 reps)<br>  3. free jumps (3 sets/10 reps)<br>  4. cone hops over 10 yards (3 reps)<br>  5. lateral line jumps (45 seconds per rep/3 reps) - work:rest ratio 1:1 |
| **WEDNESDAY** | ♦ 20 minutes of aerobic work with the ball<br>♦ Agility drills:<br>  1. triangle cone drill (5 reps)<br>  2. square cone run (10 reps)<br>  3. zig zag drill over 15 yards/minimum of 9 cuts (5 reps)<br>  4. t-cone drill (5 reps) |

| Week #13 | |
|---|---|
| MONDAY | ♦ 3 mile run in less than 20 minutes<br>♦ 80 yard acceleration sprints X 10 (jog 20 yards/sprint 60 yards = 1 rep)<br>♦ 14 X 40 yard sprints (sprint distance, walk back to start, repeat) (14 reps) |
| WEDNESDAY | ♦ 2 mile run under 12 minutes 15 seconds |
| FRIDAY | ♦ 20 minute run for maximum distance (record distance)<br>♦ Hill running X 10 reps (run up 5 hills facing forward, run up 5 hills facing backward)<br>♦ Shuttle run using 20 yard boundaries (5 reps)<br>♦ Jump rope 5 minutes<br>♦ Plyometics: box jumps (20 reps/4 sets) |

| Week #14 | |
|---|---|
| MONDAY | ♦ 80 yard acceleration sprints X 16 reps (20 yards at $^1/_2$ speed - 20 yards and $^3/_4$ speed - 40 yards at full speed)<br>♦ 10 yard sprints X 20 reps<br>♦ Agility drills:<br>  1. carrioca over 20 yards (10 reps)<br>  2. sprint/shuffle/sprint over 30 yards (5 reps)<br>♦ Plyometrics:<br>  1. skate bounding over 20 yards (10 reps)<br>  2. double leg bounding over 10 yards (10 reps)<br>  3. quick leaps (3 reps/30 seconds per rep) |
| WEDNESDAY | ♦ 2 mile run under 12:00 minutes |
| FRIDAY | ♦ 60 yard sprints X 16 reps (sprint - walk back to start - sprint)<br>♦ 10 yard sprints X 20 reps<br>♦ Agility drills:<br>  1. 5 cone box drill (5 reps)<br>  2. t-cone drill (5 reps)<br>  3. triangle cone drill (5 reps)<br>♦ Plyometrics:<br>  1. tuck jumps with heel kick (3 sets/10 reps)<br>  2. lateral hops over distance (10 cones/3 sets)<br>  3. cone hops over distance (10 cones/3 sets)<br>  4. depth jumps (3 sets/10 reps) |

| Week #15 | |
|---|---|
| **MONDAY** | ♦ 2 mile run under 12 minutes<br>♦ 15 minutes of agility drills<br>♦ 15 minutes of plyometrics |
| **WEDNESDAY** | ♦ 30 minutes of aerobic work with the ball<br>♦ 20 minutes of sprint work |
| **FRIDAY** | Off day |
| **SATURDAY** | Preseason training begins |

# Bibliography

Chyzowych, Walter. *The Official Soccer Book*. Chicago: Rand
    McNally, 1979

deVries, Herbert. *Physiology of Exercise*. Dubuque:
    William C. Brown Co., 1980

Ekblom, Bjorn. *Football (Soccer): Handbook of Sports Medi-
    cine and Science*. London: Blackwell Scientific Publica-
    tions, 1994

Fox, Edward, and Mathews, Donald. *The Physiological Basis
    of Physical Education and Athletics (3rd edition)*. New
    York: CBS College Publishing, 1981

Henshaw, Richard. *The Encyclopedia of World Soccer*. Wash-
    ington, D.C: New Republic Books, 1979

Luxbacher, Joseph A. *Soccer: Steps to Success*. Champaign: Human Kinetics, 1991

Luxbacher, Joseph A. *Soccer: Winning Techniques*. Dubuque: Eddie Bowers Publishing, 1992

Luxbacher, Joseph A. *The Soccer Goalkeeper*. Champaign: Human Kinetics, 1993

Luxbacher, Joseph A. *Soccer Practice Games*. Champaign: Human Kinetics, 1995

Nike Research Review. *Nike Sport Research Laboratory, Volume No. 5*, 1997

Pearl, Bill. *Getting Stronger*. California: Shelter Publications, 1986

Schum, Tim. *Coaching Soccer*. Indianaplis: Masters Press, 1996

Sharkey, Brian J. *Fitness and Health*. Champaign, II: Human Kinetics, 1997

# About the Author

Joe Luxbacher is the men's soccer coach at the University of Pittsburgh. A former professional player in the North American Soccer League (NASL) and Major Indoor Soccer League (MISL), Joe has more than 30 years of experience playing and coaching soccer at all levels. He holds an "A" Coaching License from the United States Soccer Federation, and was 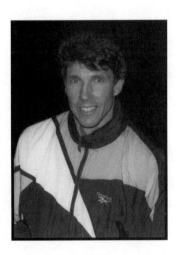 named the Big East conference soccer coach of the year in 1992 and again in 1995. Joe was selected for the Beadling Soccer Club Hall of Fame in 1995. He has authored ten books and more than 90 magazine articles on sport and fitness-related topics, and presently serves as the Fitness Editor of *Total Health Magazine.*

Coach Luxbacher holds a Ph.D. from the University of Pittsburgh with a specialization in the Management and Administration of Physical Education and Athletics. Since 1978 he has served as the director and president of Keystone Soccer Kamps and has offered educational soccer camps and clinics to thousands of youth players and coaches. He also directs the Shoot to Score soccer camp programs that focus on the skills and tactics needed to finish the attack.

Joe, his wife Gail, and their daughter Eliza live in Pittsburgh where they enjoy a variety of outdoor pursuits, including photography, hiking and canoeing.